In the Beginning

IN THE BEGINNING

Readings on Infancy

Edited by Jay Belsky

New York Columbia University Press 1982

Library of Congress Cataloging in Publication Data
Main entry under title:

In the beginning.

Bibliography: p.
Includes index.
1. Infant psychology—Addresses, essays, lectures. I. Belsky, Jay, 1952–
[DNLM: 1. Child psychology—Essays. WS 105 I35]
BF719.I52 155.4'22 81-10008
ISBN 0-231-05114-X AACR2
ISBN 0-231-05115-8 (pbk.)

Columbia University Press
New York Guildford, Surrey

Printed in the United States of America
Clothbound editions of Columbia University Press books are
Smyth-sewn and printed on permanent and durable acid-free paper.

Contents

Acknowledgments

The editor would like to thank the following publishers for permission to reprint materials used in this book. It should be noted that, to achieve uniformity, we have in some cases slightly altered the original reference and/or footnote formats to conform with the author-date method of citation used throughout this book. It was also necessary to make some editorial changes appropriate to an anthology of this kind.

"Human Babies as Embryos" by S. J. Gould: From *Natural History*, 85:22–26, 1976. Used with permission from *Natural History*, April, 1980. Copyright © American Museum of Natural History, 1976.

"Transactional Models of Early Social Relations" by A. Sameroff. From *Human Development* 18:65–79, 1975. Used with permission from S. Karger AG, Arnold-Bocklin Strasse.

"The Coherence of Individual Development" by L. A. Sroufe. From *American Psychologist* 34:834–841, 1979. Copyright © (1979) by the American Psychological Association. Reprinted by permission.

"Smoking During Pregnancy" by A. Landesman-Dwyer. From *Teratology* 19:119–125, 1979. Used with permission from Wistar Press.

From Streissguth, A. "Maternal Alcoholism and the Outcome of Pregnancy." In M. Greenblatt (Ed.), *Alcohol Problems in Women and Children*, 1977. Reprinted by permission of Grove and Stratton, Inc. and the author.

"Lasting Behavioral Effects of Obstetrical Medication on Children: Research Findings and Public Policy Implications" by Y. Brackbill. From Steward and Steward (Eds.), *Compulsory Hospitalization or Freedom of Choice in Childbirth?* 3 Vols., Marble Hill, MO:NAPSAC, 2nd printing, 1980, pp. 167–168.

"Parent-to-Infant Bonding" by M. Klaus and J. Kennell. From *Recent Advances in Pediatrics* No. 5, edited by David Hull. Copyright © 1976 by Churchill Livingstone, New York. Used with permission from Churchill Livingstone.

"Prematurity: Effects in Parent-Infant Interaction" by S. Goldberg. From *Journal of Pediatric Psychology*, 1978, *3*, 137–144. Used by permission from Plenum Publishing Co.

"Perinatal Indicators and Psychophysiological Precursors of Crib Death" by L. Lipsitt. From *Early Developmental Hazards: Predictors and Precautions*, edited by F. Forowitz. Copyright © 1978 by Westview Press. Used with permission from Westview Press.

"Our Developing Knowledge of Infant Perception and Cognition" by L. Cohen. From *American Psychologist* 34:894–898, 1979. Copyright © (1977) by the American Psychological Association. Reprinted by permission.

"Transition in Infant Sensorimotor Development and the Prediction of Childhood IW" by R. McCall, P. Hogarty, and N. Hurlburt. From *American Psychologist* 27:728–748, 1972. Copyright © (1976) by the American Psychological Association. Reprinted by permission.

"From exploration to play: A cross-sectional study of infant free play" by Jay Belsky and Robert K. Most. From *Developmental Psychology*, 1981, in press. Copyright © 1981 by the American Psychological Association. Reprinted by Permission.

"The Development of Infant-Mother Attachment" by M. Ainsworth. Reprinted from *Review of Child Development*, Vol. 3, by B. Caldwell and H. Riciutti, Editors. By permission of University of Chicago Press, 1974.

"Continuity and Adaptation in the Second Year: The Relationship Between Quality of Attachment and Later Competence" by L. Matas, R. Arend, and L. Sroufe. From *Child Development* 49:547–556, 1978. Used with permission from The Society for Research in Child Development.

"Self, Other and Fear: The Reactions of Infants to People" by M. Lewis and J. Brooks-Gunn. Paper presented at the Eastern Psychological Association meetings, Boston, April, 1972. Copyright © 1972 by M. Lewis and J. Brooks-Gunn. Used with permission from authors.

"Growth of Social Play with Peers During the Second Year of Life" by C. Eckerman, J. Whatley, and S. Kutz. From *Developmental Psy-*

chologist 11:42–49, 1975. Copyright © (1975) by the American Psychological Association. Reprinted by permission.

"Dimensions of Early Stimulation and Their Differential Effects on Infant Development" by L. Yarrow, J. Rubenstein, F. Pedersen, & J. Janowski. From *Merrill-Palmer Quarterly* 18:205–218, 1972. Used with permission from The Merrill-Palmer Institute.

"Infant Obedience and Maternal Behavior: The Origins of Socialization Reconsidered" by D. Stayton, R. Hogan, M. Ainsworth. From *Child Development* 42:1057–1069, 1971. Used with permission from The Society for Research in Child Development.

"And Daddy Makes Three: The Father's Impact on Mother and Young Child" by K. A. Clarke-Stewart. From *Child Development* 49:466–478, 1978. Used with permission from The Society for Research in Child Development.

"Mother, Father, Infant as an Interactive System" by F. Pedersen. Paper presented at the annual meetings of the American Psychological Association, Chicago, September, 1975.

"Interactions Between 18-Month-Olds and Their Preschool-Age Siblings" by M. Lamb. From *Child Development* 49:51–54, 1978. Used with permission from The Society for Research in Child Development.

"Maternal Employment and Mother Child Interaction" by S. Cohen. From *Merrill-Palmer Quarterly* 24:189–197, 1978. Used with permission from the Merrill-Palmer Institute.

"The Effects of Day Care: A Critical Review" by J. Belsky and L. Steinberg. From *Child Development* 49:924–929, 1978. Used with permission from The Society for Research in Child Development.

"Compensatory Education for Disadvantaged Children" by C. Raney and C. Campbell. From *School Review* 87:171–189, 1979. Used with permission from University of Chicago Press.

In the Beginning

Introduction

Every long journey begins with the first step. And so it is with the life span, the first step being the period of infancy. While many today debate the significance of early experience for later development and whether or not the child is truly the father of the man, there are those of us who remain convinced that the first stage of life is not only important for subsequent development but is also fascinating in its own right and revealing of developmental principles that function across the life span.

It is from these starting points, or basic assumptions, that this volume emerged. My purpose in planning this book was to collect a series of theoretical essays, empirical studies, and critical reviews of research which document these themes and, in so doing, illustrate the explosion in understanding that has taken place in the last decade concerning the first stage of life. This book begins, then, with a series of essays which highlight general themes that recur throughout the volume—specifically, the unique circumstances and developmental plasticity of human infancy, transactional processes in early experience, and continuity in development.

Following the section on general themes, a developmental framework is adhered to, which leads us to consider first prenatal and then perinatal influences on infant functioning. As I believe these essays demonstrate, the quality of individual development may be circumscribed by the very nature of these early experiences. Indeed, in some cases, we must regard the human fetus and neonate as a victim of circumstances. This is not to say that what happens during the beginning of life fully determines what will come later, but, nevertheless, it can be extremely influential. In fact, one of the most interesting questions that the study of infancy raises, and that several readings in this volume consider, concerns the conditions that maintain or alter developmental trajectories established during any developmental epoch.

In the third and fourth sections, a less chronological and more substantively analytic framework is adopted to examine first cognitive-perceptual development and then socioemotional development during the first two years of life. Let it be said now, even if it is to be repeated later, that this division of psychological development is artificial, as the human organism in an integrated whole. We divide him up for heuristic purposes only.

Having examined very early experience in the womb and in the perinatal period, and having inquired into intellectual and social development, attention is turned in the fifth section of this book to postnatal influences—both within the family and beyond—on infant functioning. Here I have tried to select articles that document the significance of all nuclear family members—mothers, fathers, and siblings—to the infant, and discuss several contemporary issues that affect infant growth and development, specifically day care and maternal employment.

The knowledge that studies of early experience and infant development generates is, for many of us, a means to an end; that end being efforts to facilitate and enhance development. And it is in early intervention efforts, two of which are described in the final section, that the need for basic science becomes so evident to those concerned with supporting the development of children growing up under less than optimal circumstances (e.g., in poverty). In essence, then, one can regard much of the work covered in the earlier sections as a necessary prelude to the work described in the final section. It is my hope that the reader will come to recognize the essential harmony that can exist between what are often called basic science and applied science and regarded all to frequently as oppositional approaches to the study of development.

In selecting and editing these articles, I have tried to keep at the forefront of my thoughts the prospective reader. As I envision this volume, it is primarily a resource for undergraduates, although it could clearly be used in certain graduate courses. However, the graduate student and instructor should be aware that certain scientific details (e.g., interobserver reliabilities, statistical tests) have been eliminated from many reports so that, at least for the novice scientist, the forest is not lost for the trees. This principle has guided my editing not only of the sections on empirical studies dealing with methodology and statistical analysis, but also of the discussions of background research and conceptual issues. Throughout the process of preparing this book, I continually strived to make the principal themes of each reading evident by eliminating sections that I felt sidetracked the primary discussion. I trust I have not violated the integrity of any manuscript in exercising this editorial liberty.

To facilitate the instructor's decision in selecting readings from this volume when the entire book is not be be studied, I have prepared introductions to each of the six major sections. In these I have tried to make explicit what I consider to be the major contribution of each selection and, thus, my reasons for including it here. I have also attempted to explain the reasoning that lies behind the ordering of papers within a section, for I have endeavored to relate the essays so that each follows logically from the one that preceded it and leads to the next. To the extent that I have succeeded in this task, the whole of this volume will be greater than the sum of its parts.

PART I

General Themes

To many observers, what makes human beings so unique as a species is their plasticity or ability to change and adapt to the contexts in which they live. This remarkable flexibility, it has been argued, derives from the very first stage of life, for infancy is a period when the young, dependent, and relatively helpless human organism experiences learning opportunities unlike those of any other animal. Stephen Jay Gould, a paleontologist, reports in the first paper in this volume that these special opportunities for learning are themselves by-products of a unique gestational pattern which sets the prenatal experience of humans apart from other mammals. While altricial mammals have brief gestations and give birth to large litters of poorly developed young with limited social skills, and while precocial mammals have long gestations and give birth to a few well-developed and socially skilled babies, humans display neither of these reproductive strategies in its entirety. Instead, while we share many precocial characteristics with our primate cousins, including long life spans, large brains, and small litters, our babies are also like altricial animals—helpless and undeveloped at birth. In sum, Gould argues that human babies are born early, that is, while still in the embryonic state.

The reason for this early expulsion from the womb is to be found in the physical demands of childbearing and the genius of evolutionary programming. Given the large size of the human brain at birth, mothers would be unable to deliver a child much past the standard gestation period and still survive. The birth canal would simply not tolerate a much larger skull. Consequently, the human baby is born while brain growth is still in progress. And the fact that the brain continues to develop postnatally, while the organism is exposed to a complex environment, creates the possibility for the early learning of which we spoke earlier. Without this period of early learning, our plasticity as a species would be severely limited and, as a consequence, so would our achievements, especially our uncanny ability to successfully adapt to the myriad of contexts in which human development takes place.

It is a truism in the scientific community today that this development is neither a product of nature (e.g., genes, biology, maturation) nor nurture (i.e., experience), but rather of the interaction of these two domains of influence. In the second paper in this volume, "Transactional Models of Early Social Relations," Sameroff underscores this point in noting that, in the case of the human infant, nature and nurture are contributors to the developmental process and only through their dynamic interplay can they be said to determine the course of infant growth and change. Exactly how such growth and change take place is of critical importance to students of human development, for it represents a concern for the *process* by which development occurs rather than for that all-too-frequent focus of psychological research, the *outcomes* of development (e.g., intelligence, achievement). And it is this issue of process which Sameroff concerns himself with in detailing the transactional nature of the infant's experience in the world. By directing attention to the mutual, constant give-and-take between organism and environment, Sameroff's article gives substance to the abstract conception of nature-nurture interaction. As he says, "Practically speaking, the infant is affecting his caretaking environment at the same time the caretaking environment is affecting the infant." The dynamic system's properties of the infant and his caregiver(s) must be appreciated, then, if the course of development is to be understood.

What, though, are the consequences of this interplay between caregiver and infant and, more generally, of development during the infant years? At a time when increasing numbers of scholars question the developmental significance of infancy (the first stage of postnatal life) and the notion of continuity in development (i.e., "the child as the father of the man"), Sroufe argues, in his paper entitled "The Coherence of Individual Development," that a smoothly synchronized mother-infant system not only fosters the secure emotional attachment of infant to caregiver but, in so doing, lays the foundation for competent functioning in the postinfancy years. The key to understanding the coherence of development, he maintains, lies in the recognition that "psychological development is characterized, not by mere additions, but by transformations and epigenesis," that is, by lawful change.

In detailing the principles of a theory of individual development, Sroufe underscores the necessity of appreciating the salient issues of each ontogenic epoch and of examining the total functioning of the developing organism rather than individual behaviors that the organism displays. Such an approach to the study of continuity in development should not only reveal the qualitative changes the individual undergoes, but also the significance of infancy as the beginning of the life span. Sroufe does not imply, however, that what transpires during the first stage of postnatal life determines, in any simplistic manner, the course of subsequent development, but only that this period of growth and change will exert some influence. Given the dynamic nature of the developmental process, exactly what that influence will be will depend upon the subsequent transactions of the ever-changing organism with the ever-changing environment in which it lives. To a significant degree, the nature of such transactions will be affected by what the organism brings to these encounters. And here, of course, lies the significance of infancy. Like each subsequent period of development, the period of infancy will not determine future growth and change, but will nevertheless influence it.

In sum, then, these first three articles introduce three general themes that will recur throughout this volume: (1) the extended dependency period of the human infant and the opportunity this offers for early learning; (2) the bidirectional nature of caregiver-infant influence; and (3) the significance of infancy for later development.

1

Human Babies as Embryos

STEPHEN JAY GOULD

In the November 1975 issue of *Natural History*, my friend Bob Martin wrote a piece on strategies of reproduction in primates. He focused upon the work of one of my favorite scientists—the idiosyncratic Swiss zoologist Adolf Portmann. In his voluminous studies, Portmann has identified two basic patterns in the reproductive strategies of mammals. Some mammals, usually designated by us as "primitive," have brief gestations and give birth to large litters of poorly developed young (tiny, hairless, helpless, and with unopened eyes and ears). Life spans are short, brains are small (relative to body size), and social behaviors are not well developed. Portmann refers to this pattern as altricial. On the other hand, many "advanced" mammals have long gestations, long life spans, big brains, complex social behavior, and give birth to a few, well-developed babies capable, at least in part, of fending for themselves at birth. These traits mark the precocial mammals. In Portmann's vision of evolution as a process leading inexorably upward to greater spiritual development, the altricial pattern is primitive and preparatory to the higher precocial type that evolves along with enlarged brains. Most English-speaking evolutionists would reject this interpretation and link the basic patterns to immediate requirements of different modes of life. (I have often used this column to vent my own prejudices against equating evolution with "progress.") The altricial pattern, Martin argues, seems to correlate with marginal, fluctuating, and unstable environments in which animals do best by making as many offspring as they possibly can—so that some can weather the harshness of the climate or the uncertainty of resources. The precocial pattern fits better with stable, tropical environments. Here, with more predictable resources, animals can invest their limited energy in a few well-developed offspring.

Whatever the explanation, no one will deny that primates are the archetypical precocial mammals. Relative to body sizes, their brains are the biggest and their gestation times and life spans are the longest among mammals. Litter sizes, in most cases, have been reduced to the absolute minimum of one. Babies are well-developed and capable at birth. However, although Martin doesn't mention it, we encounter one obviously glaring and embarrassing exception—namely, us. We share most of the precocial characters with our primate cousins—long life, large brains, and small litters—but our babies are as helpless and undeveloped at birth as those of most primitive altricial mammals. In fact, Portmann himself refers to human babies as "secondarily altricial." Why did this most precocial of all species in some traits (notably the brain) evolve a baby far less developed and more helpless than that of its primate ancestors?

I will propose an answer to this question that is bound to strike most readers as patently absurd: Human babies are born as embryos, and embryos they remain for about the first nine months of life. If women gave birth when they "should"—after a gestation of about a year and a half—our babies would share the standard precocial features of other primates. This is Portmann's position, developed in a series of German articles during the 1940s and essentially unknown in this country. Ashley Montagu reached the same conclusion independently in a paper published in the *Journal of the American Medical Association* in October 1961. Oxford psychologist R. E. Passingham has championed it in a piece published in 1975 in the technical journal *Brain, Behavior and Evolution*. I also cast my lot with this select group in regarding the argument as basically correct.

The initial impression that such an argument can only be arrant nonsense arises from the length of human gestation. Gorillas and chimps may not be far behind, but human gestation is still the longest among primates. How then can I claim that human neonates are embryos because they are born (in some sense) too soon? The answer is that planetary days may not provide an appropriate measure of time in all biological calculations. Some questions can only be treated properly when time is measured relatively in terms of an animal's own metabolism or developmental rate. For example, we know that mammalian life spans vary from a few weeks to more than a century. But is this a "real" distinction in terms of a mammal's own perception of time and rate? Does a rat really live "less" than an elephant? Laws of scaling dictate that small, warm-blooded animals live at a faster pace than larger relatives. The heart beats more rapidly and metabolism proceeds at a greatly elevated rate. In fact, for several criteria of relative time, all mammals live about the same amount. All, for example, breathe about the same number of times during their lives (small, short-lived mammals breathe more rapidly than larger, slow metabolizers).

In astronomical days, human gestation is long, but relative to human developmental rates, it is truncated and abbreviated. In my column for *Natural History* in May 1975, I argued that a (if not the) major feature of human evolution has been the marked slowing up of our development. Our brains grow more slowly and for a longer time than those of other primates, our bones ossify much later and the period of our childhood is greatly extended. In fact, we never reach the levels of development attained by most primates. Human adults retain, in several important respects, the juvenile traits of ancestral primates—an evolutionary phenomenon called neoteny. Neoteny has been crucial in human evolution for two reasons:

1. It provides a morphology adapted to our mode of life. We have a large brain because rapid fetal growth rates continue in humans long after they have ceased in other primates. Our bulbous cranium and short face resemble those of juvenile primates, not those of low-browed, long-faced primate adults. We can stand erect because our foramen magnum—the hole in our skull for attachment with the vertebral column—lies under our brain, not behind it as in four-footed mammals. The foramen magnum of fetal

primates (and other mammals) lies under the brain, but migrates back during development.

2. The slow rate of our development has been important in itself, quite apart from the juvenile morphology that it permits us to retain as adults. We are primarily learning animals; we need a long period of dependent and flexible childhood to provide time for the cultural transmission that makes us human. If we matured and began to fend for ourselves as early as most other mammals, we would never develop the mental capacity that our neotenic brain permits.

Compared with other primates, we grow and develop at a snail's pace; yet our gestation period is but a few days longer than that of gorillas and chimpanzees. Relative to our own developmental rate, our gestation has been markedly shortened. If length of gestation had slowed down as much as the rest of our growth and development, human babies would be born anywhere from seven to eight months (Passingham's estimate) to a year (Portmann and Ashley Montagu's estimate) after the nine months actually spent *in utero*.

But am I not indulging in mere metaphor or trick of phrase in designating the human baby as "still an embryo"? I have just raised two children of my own past this tender age, and have experienced all the joy and mystery of their mental and physical development—things that could never happen in a dark, confining womb. Still, I side with Portmann when I consider the data on their physical growth, for during their first year, human babies share the growth patterns of primate and mammalian fetuses, not of other primate babies. (The identification of certain growth patterns as either fetal or postnatal is not arbitrary. Postnatal development is not a mere prolongation of fetal tendencies; birth is a time of marked discontinuity in many features.) Human neonates, for example, have not yet ossified the ends of limb bones or fingers; ossification centers are usually entirely absent in the finger bones of newborn humans. This level of ossification corresponds to the eighteenth fetal week of macaque monkeys. When macaques are born at 24 weeks, their limb bones are ossified to an extent not reached by humans until years after birth. More crucially, our brains continue to grow at rapid, fetal rates after birth. The brains of most mammals are essentially fully formed at birth. Other primates extend brain development into early postnatal growth. Macaque brains are 65 percent complete at birth, chimpanzee brains, 40.5 percent. The brain of a human baby is only 23 percent of its final size at birth. Brains of chimps and gorillas reach 70 percent of final size early in the first year; we do not attain this value until early in our third year. Passingham writes, "Man's brain does not reach the proportion found for the chimpanzee at birth until around 6 months after birth. This time corresponds quite well with the time at which man would be expected to be born if this gestation period were as high a proportion of his development and life span as it is in apes."

A.H. Schultz, probably the greatest primate anatomist of the century, summarized his comparative study of growth in primates by stating, "It is evident that human ontogeny is not unique in regard to the duration of life in utero, but that it has become highly specialized in the striking postponement of the completion of growth and of the onset of senility."

But why are human babies born before their time? Why has evolution extended our general development so greatly, but held our gestation time in check, thereby giving us an essentially embryonic baby? Why was gestation not equally prolonged with the rest of development? In Portmann's spiritual view of evolution, this precocious birth must be a function of mental requirements. He argues that humans, as learning animals, need to leave the dark, unchallenging womb to gain access, as flexible embryos, to the rich extrauterine environment of sights, smells, sounds, and touches.

But I believe (along with Ashley Montagu and Passingham) that a more important reason lies in a consideration that Portmann dismisses contemptuously as coarsely mechanical and materialistic. From what I have seen (although I cannot know for sure), human birth is a joyful experience when properly rescued from arrogant male physicians who seem to want total control over a process they cannot experience. Nenetheless, I do not think it can be denied that human birth is difficult compared with that of most other mammals. To put it rather grossly, it's a tight squeeze. We know that female primates can die in attempted childbirth when fetal heads are too large to pass through the pelvic canal. A. H. Schultz illustrates the stillborn fetus of a hamadryas baboon and the pelvic canal of its dead mother; the embryo's head is a good deal larger than the canal. Schultz concludes that fetal size is near its limit in this species: "While selection undoubtedly tends to favor large diameters of the female pelvis, it must also act against any prolongation of gestation or at least against unduly large newborns."

There are not, I am confident, many human females who could give birth successfully to a year-old-baby.

The culprit in this tale is our most important evolutionary specialization, our large brain. In most mammals, brain growth is entirely a fetal phenomenon. But since the brain never gets very large, this poses no problem for birth. In larger-brained monkeys, growth is delayed somewhat to permit postnatal enlargement of the brain, but relative times of gestation need not be altered. Human brains, however, are so large that another strategy must be added for successful birth—gestation must be shortened relative to general development, and birth must occur when the brain is only one-fourth its final size.

Our brain has probably reached the end of its increase in size. The paramount trait of our evolution has finally limited its own potential for future growth. Barring some radical redesign of the female pelvis, we will have to make do with the brains we have if we want to be born at all. But, no matter. We can happily spend the next several millennia learning what to do with an immense potential that we have scarcely begun to understand or exploit.

2

Transactional Models in Early Social Relations

ARNOLD SAMEROFF

Mechanistic orientations to the study of human development have focussed on a search for variables in either the organism or the environment which will be predictive of the individual's later behavior. While increasing sophistication in scientific circles has permitted a redefinition of the nature-nurture question from an either-or to an interactive model, this interactive model is still lacking by its failure to consider the transactions between organism and environment which result in their mutual alteration throughout development.

Sameroff and Chandler (1975) have described three models for understanding the developmental consequences of early trauma—a main effects model, an interactional model, and a transactional model. In the main effects model, either constitution or environment is considered to be the sole contributor to later developmental outcomes. On the constitution side, for example, mental retardation might be attributed to minimal brain damage resulting from birth complications, or schizophrenia might be attributed to genetic transmission. On the environmental side, these same disorders could be attributed to impoverished child-rearing surroundings or to a schizophrenogenic mother.

When the evidence for these main effects models are evaluated, linear chains of efficient causality are not found. In general, children with delivery complications do not become retarded nor do offspring of schizophrenics become schizophrenic. In specific, those children with early trauma who later do show signs of deviancy also have had deviant child-rearing experiences. In the case of children who have had complicated births, those growing up in middle-class homes with educated parents who are emotionally stable show no later signs of deviancy related to the early trauma. However, infants with the same complications who are raised in families of lower socioeconomic status, or with uneducated parents, or with emotionally disturbed parents show many behavioral deviancies later on.

These findings have led investigators to reject the main effects model and adopt instead an interactional one in which both constitution and environment must be taken into consideration. A table can be set up in which each combination of constitution and environment is assigned a developmental consequence. Children with good constitutions raised in good environments will have the best outcomes. Children with poor constitutions raised in inadequate environments will have the worse outcomes. Children with good constitutions raised in poor environments or poor constitutions raised in good environments will have intermediate outcomes.

The interactional model certainly is an advance over the main effects model in terms of predictive efficiency, but it still leaves much unexplained variance both practically and theoretically. Practically, many children grow up in the worst possible situation, yet achieve greatness, while, conversely, children with no identifiable constitutional problem raised in the best of environments show serious later deviancies. Theoretically, predictive efficiency is not the same as knowledge of the processes by which development takes place. The interactional model makes the assumption that good or bad constitutions or environments can be defined independently of each other and that these evaluations will persist over time. The mechanistic overtones of both the main effects model and the interactional model are clear in the way in which the two aspects—nature and nurture—are viewed as elements whose structure is constant over time.

To give a full role to the variety of effects found between and within constitutional and environmental variables, a model is necessary which can deal with the processes as well as the outcomes of development. Such a model has been proposed by Sameroff and Chandler (1975), which they have labeled the *transactional* model. Its characteristics are implicit in any organismic approach to developmental phenomenon and has been described by others under various titles, e.g., Riegel's (1972, 1975) citation of Rubinstein's double-interaction model. The underlying assumptions of the *transactional* model are that the contact between organism and environment is a transaction in which each is altered by the other. Practically speaking, the infant is affecting his caretaking environment at the same time that the caretaking environment is affecting the infant.

Mother-Infant Transactions

The focus on developmental transactions in social relations has been growing over the past decade. Bell (1968) explored the literature on the direction of effects in the early caretaking situation. He argued that seeing children as passive recipients of environmental inputs fits only a one-sided model of parental determination of behavior. Many studies demonstrated that the child may be strongly involved in determining the nature of his early social relationships. In many situations parental behaviors can be seen not to be spontaneously emitted but rather to be elicited by the child's characteristics and behavior.

The ethologists have focused on the eliciting properties of the infant on parental behavior, but, following their own mechanistic bent, ethologists have defined these behaviors as innate, genetically programed activities and features which are not altered by environmental consequences (Eibl-Eibesfeldt 1970). Rosenblatt (1970), invoking a concept of behavioral synchrony, has been able to demonstrate how the changing characteristics of the infant rat initiate and maintain maternal behavior which then alters the behavior of the infant. Rosenblatt's excellent reports of synchronous transactions in infant-parent rat pairs are far superior to any descriptions of similar human pairings.

Thomas, Chess, & Brich (1968) gave strong support to the need for a dynamic, process-oriented theory of development in their studies of infant temperament. They were able to differentiate 'constitutional' differences in the temperaments of three-month-old infants. Given parents with similar attitudes and backgrounds, infants with different temperaments elicited different caretaking reactions and, as a consequence, had differing developmental outcomes. Most important, the developmental outcomes for these infants were not implicit in the child but were a result of the different caretaking behaviors the child elicited from the parent. In other words, the child's developmental outcome was a function of the dynamic system properties of the infant, together with his caretaking environment, rather than a function of either the infant or caretaker alone. The obvious need in research with early human social relations are analyses of such transactions. The properties of the human newborn which elicit parenting behavior must be evaluated in conjunction with the effects on the child of the behavior which he elicits.

3

The Coherence of Individual Development

Early Care, Attachment, and Subsequent Developmental Issues

L. ALAN SROUFE

The idea that the child is a coherent person, that despite changes he or she remains in important ways the same individual, has been a powerful force in developmental psychology. In many ways it spurred the emergence of our field, and it moves us forward still. For if the child is a coherent person and individual development a coherent process, and if conditions can be specified that promote psychologically healthy or unhealthy development, then there are powerful implications not only for behavioral scientists but for our entire society. If, for example, one's feelings of self-worth and personal power (efficacy), one's expectations concerning people, and one's capacity for empathic involvement with others are strongly influenced by early experience, then we cannot hesitate to examine fully our public policies in these times of rapid social change. The type and extent of out-of-home care become more than purely economic matters. Teenage pregnancy, chemical dependency, physical or sexual abuse of children, and other signs of family dysfunction become matters of urgent national concern. It becomes clear that nothing is more important than understanding the shaping of the child.

Only recently, however, has continuity in individual development proved empirically demonstrable. This was despite the fact that such an assumption is central in prominent developmental theories and despite the fact that intuition and personal experience testified daily to the coherence of the individual. Research, so it seemed, previously suggested that such continuity was an illusion. But it was the research that was wrong, not the idea of continuity.

One problem in past research on continuity concerned errors of measurement. Measuring behavioral continuity in the developing child is difficult because behaviors that are beyond the capacity of the younger infant are added rapidly to the repertoire, old behaviors take on new meanings, and behavior becomes organized in increasingly complex ways. Its meaning varies with the behavioral and situational context. Therefore, behavior of children must be assessed extensively across situations or in especially salient situations. Counting frequencies of particular behaviors in a single observational session or examining children's performances on a single task cannot yield stable individual differences any more than can performance on a single item from an intelligence test (Epstein 1979). Unless measurements are stable, individuals cannot reveal their continuities.

Another problem in research on continuity is conceptual. Psychological development is characterized not by mere additions but by transformations and epigenesis. Infants are not merely small children. Therefore, one cannot find continuity by simply measuring the same behavior over time. "Clingy" overdependency, for example, is one form of maladaptation in the preschool years. Such dependency in the norm in infancy. Recent studies have shown that infants who, when threatened or distressed, actively seek physical contact with the caregiver, and who cling to the caregiver and derive comfort from such contact (i.e., are effectively dependent), become effectively autonomous as toddlers and competent as preschoolers (Arend, Gove, &

Sroufe 1979; Main 1977; Matas, Arend, & Sroufe 1978; Waters, Wippman, & Sroufe 1979).

Development does not proceed in a linear, incremental manner. Not only are capacities added; there are changes in behavioral organization. Through such change the infant is transformed, becoming qualitatively different in the way it views and transacts with the world. Periods of reorganization can be defined, with consequent changes in focal development issues. Assessment of individual differences should address these changing issues.

The Child as Active Participant in Its Own Experience

To understand the coherence of individual adaptation, viewing children as active participants in their own experience is essential. At least by the second half year, the infant's reaction to events is subjective; it is determined by evaluative processes within the infant, as well as by objective information. Individual infants and children differ in their tendencies to see events as opportunities or threats, in their threshold for threat, in their capacity to maintain organized behavior in the face of arousal (novelty, complexity), and in their ability to derive security from the presence of the caregiver. More generally, children vary in their abilities to draw on personal and environmental resources in the face of a challenge.

Normative studies of infant development illustrate the role of subjective factors in behavior. The same event can produce strikingly different reactions depending on its context. For example, mother putting on a mask uniformly elicits smiling and laughter in a playful home context. In the laboratory, however, following a separation experience, the same masked approach by the mother produces almost no smiling. Some infants become distressed, especially if a masked stranger approaches first. With groups of subjects, any reaction can be produced by varying familiarization time, setting, sequence of events, and availability of the caregiver (Sroufe, Waters, & Matas 1974).

The reactions cannot be due to novelty per se. The event is novel in every case (and less so following the stranger). Nor can the reaction be due simply to amount of arousal. High levels of arousal are required for laughter as well as for distress. And even if one fully calms an infant following separation (he returns to play and autonomic levels recover), the negative effect of the separation is still produced when the mother subsequently puts on the mask. Apparently the infant's threshold for threat (the amount of arousal tolerable) has been altered. On the other hand, in the playful home context, the most arousing play (e.g., mother bouncing the infant) rarely leads to distress. No fixed amount of arousal automatically leads to distress. Infants can stay engaged and affectively positive, even purposefully repeat the event, when highly aroused.

Individual children elicit different reactions from the environment; they also differentially seek, filter, interpret, and evaluate experience. The infant who cannot separate from mother to explore the novel playroom and the preschooler who isolates himself from peers are not having the same experience as the more positively engaged child. Once constitution and early experience have interacted to produce the emergent personality, the child is an active force in his or her own development. As Adler wrote, the child is the artist as well as the painting. Personality develops from a foundation, increasing in organizational complexity, differentiating from early general modes of engaging the environment. Later reorganizations are elaborations and transformations of this foundation. It is for this reason that the quality of early experience, especially of significant relationships, is of fundamental importantce in development.

Early Developmental Issues

To trace the course of healthy development we must be able to assess qualitative differences in functioning among children at different points in time, from early environmental transactions within the caregiver-infant relationship to later functioning outside the home. In this task it is useful to view development as organized around a series of issues. Learning to manage tension and active exploration have already been mentioned; other issues are also important. A working scheme is presented in table 3.1. Parallels between this sequence and those of Piaget, Sander, and Spitz have been described elsewhere (Sroufe 1977, 1978, 1979). These issues are not viewed as tasks to be passed or failed, never to be faced again. All but the first, in fact, are lifetime psychological issues. The issues form a sequence, however, that is ascendant during various phases of early development and that lays the groundwork for approaching subsequent issues. At the same time, preceding issues are continually reworked when facing later issues. As Erikson (1963) suggested, early trust provides the foundation for autonomy, but trust is also deepened by the clarity, firmness, and support the parents provide in the autonomy phase.

The scheme can be illustrated by considering the issue for the second half year, the formation of an effective, secure attachment relationship. During this period the infant's behavior becomes focused on and organized around the caregiver. Separation protests, retreats to the caregiver when distressed, and immediate greeting reactions appear. The infant has assumed a more mutual, fully reciprocal role in interaction with the caregiver.

Attachment, of course, has its roots in earlier infancy: it is a product of caregiver-infant interaction. The infant who is secure

Table 3.1 Issues in Early Development

Phase	Age in Months	Issue	Role for caregiver
1	0–3	Physiological regulation	Smooth routines
2	3–6	Management of tension	Sensitive, cooperative interaction
3	6–12	Establishing an effective attachment relationship	Responsive availability
4	12–18	Exploration and mastery	Secure base
5	18–30	Individuation (autonomy)	Firm support
6	30–54	Management of impulses, sex role identification, peer relations	Clear roles and values, flexible self-control

in his or her attachment has experienced the caregiver as a reliable source of comforting, as responsive to his or her signals, and as available and sensitive. The infant has learned that stimulation in the context of the caregiver will generally not be overwhelming, and that when arousal threatens to exceed the infant's organizational capacity, the caregiver will intervene.

In psychoanalytic theory the caregiver's role in relieving tension is emphasized. My view emphasizes the caregiver's role in helping the infant maintain organized behavior in the face of novelty-produced excitation. In part through face-to-face play, in which the caregiver continually varies facial expression, voice tone, and movements, the infant learns to deal with novelty and complexity within a familiar context. As the caregiver engages, relaxes, then reengages the infant (all in response to the infant's signals) the infant learns to maintain organized behavior in the face of increasingly high levels of arousal (Brazelton, Kowslowski & Main 1974; Stern 1974b). There is security in that which is familiar. The attachment relationship, based on reliable patterns of interaction with the caregiver, represents security the infant can take into new situations, especially as the relationship is increasingly internalized.

Attachment has its roots in early interaction; it also lays the foundation for subsequent development. A central issue for the 12 to 18-month-old infant (phase 4) is exploration and mastery of the environment. The child who is secure in its attachment is able to use the caregiver as a base for this exploration. The mere presence of the caregiver provides sufficient security in a novel setting to promote active exploration. This psychological availability of the caregiver during exploration and later problem solving deepens the security of attachment and helps a new mode of psychological contact to evolve. The infant can be comforted by a glance across the room or by a word. At the same time, infants can affectively share their play by smiling, showing toys to the caregiver, and so forth. The infant and caregiver can remain in psychological contact, even when at a physical distance (Sroufe 1977).

Just as the quality of attachment influences the infant's exploratory competence, these early adaptations in turn influence the quality of autonomous functioning in the toddler period (Matas, Arend, & Sroufe 1978). The child who has developed mastery skills, the capacity for affective involvement, and a sense of confidence within the caregiver-infant relationship will be more enthusiastic, persistent, and effective in facing environmental challenges on its own. Later, given continued support by the caregiver, this child will be confident, skilled, and positive in dealing with peers and with tasks of the preschool period (Arend, Gove, & Sroufe 1979; Sroufe 1978). In successfully approaching each issue, the child is acquiring capacities needed for further effective adaptation.

Continuity of Individual Adaptation

When early childhood is viewed in terms of a series of organizational issues, the pursuit of the person means assessing how well the child is functioning with respect to each issue. Assessment situations, procedures, and behavioral domains tapped may be vastly different at different developmental periods; still, the prediction remains: the quality of the child's earlier adaptation will influence its adaptation with respect to subsequent issues.

We began our research on the coherence of individual adaptation with the study of infant-caregiver attachment. Ainsworth (e.g., Ainsworth et al. 1978) had provided a scheme in which attachment is viewed in terms of its balance with exploration. When stress is minimal, the securely attached child (Group B) can separate readily from the caregiver to explore. When distressed, however, by a brief separation, for example, the securely attached infant actively seeks and maintains contact until comforted, which promotes a return to play. Under other circumstances, or when the infant is older, a brief separation from the caregiver may not produce distress, especially if the baby is not left alone. If not upset, secure infants are nonetheless active in reestablishing contact, although, as noted above, the contact is interactive rather than physical.

Ainsworth described two other major patterns of attachment. One group of infants (Group A) is characterized by its avoidance (e.g., ignoring, looking or turning away from) of the caregiver upon reunion. Such avoidance is especially striking during a second reunion, when stress is presumed to be greater. Thus, although this type of infant can separate readily from its caregiver, it fails to seek contact under circumstances of need, which interferes with its return to active exploration. A third group (Group C) is characterized by its poverty of exploration and its inability to be settled upon reunion. Infants in this group may mix contact seeking with interaction resistance (squirming to get down, kicking or hitting the caregiver, or batting away offered toys) or may merely continue to cry and fuss despite attempts at comforting. (For details, see Ainsworth et al. 1978; Sroufe & Waters 1977). These patterns have been predicted by maternal behavior as early as 6–15 weeks of life.

If these individual differences do reflect emerging personality, they should forecast later functioning. To examine the consequences of these patterns of attachment, we followed up on 48 infants who were observed in a problem-solving situation when they were 2 years old. This situation was appropriate for assessing movement toward autonomous functioning (phase 5) because some of the problems were within the children's capacity and others were quite challenging (e.g., weighting down a lever with a block to raise candy from a Plexiglas box), requiring the children to fall back on the caregivers' assistance. As toddlers, securely attached infants were more enthusiastic, more persistent, and exhibited more positive affect. They complied with maternal suggestions more, ignored the mother less, and showed less oppositional behavior.

To illustrate that these patterns of adaptation have further developmental consequences for the child (away from the mother), we conducted two other studies. In the first (using data gathered by Wanda Bronson), Everett Waters and I found that quality of attachment at 15 months was related to independent Q-sort descriptions of the children in nursery school at age 3½ years. Securely attached children were later described as socially involved peer leaders who attracted the attention of others and were curious and actively engaged in their surroundings. Overall differences between securely and insecurely attached infants in "peer competence" and "personal competence" were highly significant, and these differences were not due to IQ (Waters et al. 1979).

In a more recent study we linked our work on attachment to the Blocks' important work on two dimensions of personality organization—ego control and ego resiliency (Block & Block 1979). *Ego control* refers to the degree of control the child maintains over impulses, wishes, and desires. Overcontrolled children are rigid, unable to be spontaneous; undercontrolled children cannot delay gratification, control impulses, or behave purposefully. *Ego resiliency* refers to flexibility of controls. The resilient child can plan and delay when circumstances require but can also exhibit spontaneity, enthusiasm, and curiosity, letting up controls appropriately.

We were able to obtain follow-up measures on 26 children from our original attachment study at age 5 years (Arend, Gove, & Sroufe 1979), using a subset of the Blocks' laboratory measures (e.g., Banta's curiosity box, level of aspiration, social problem solving, Lowenfeld mosaics, motor inhibition) and their observational technique. As was predicted and theoretically required, children who earlier were securely attached were independently described by their teachers as highly resilient. Items typically placed in the "most characteristic" category included "resourceful in initiating activities," "curious and exploring," and "self-reliant, confident." (Least characteristic items included "inhibited and constricted," "tends to disengage under stress," and "becomes anxious when the environment is unpredictable.") They were also described as moderate on control, neither over- nor undercontrolled. Infants classified in Groups A (avoidant) and C (resistant) were significantly lower on resiliency, with those in Group A tending to be overcontrolled, and those in Group C undercontrolled. Such patterns of over- and undercontrol already appeared incipient in the earlier attachment assessments and in our toddler data, and were in fact predicted by the Blocks. The composite laboratory data also showed the securely attached infants to be significantly higher on resiliency (laboratory battery composite and teacher Q-sort resiliency scores correlated .46, $p < .01$).

What began as a competent caregiver–infant pair led to a flexible, resourceful child. Our attachment assessments predicted later functioning more powerfully than had any previously used measures, including standardized infant tests. A focus on developmentally salient issues enables assessment that taps the core of early competence. Such predictability is not due to the inherently higher IQ of the securely attached infant or, apparently, to inborn differences in temperament, though such differences likely have important influences on behavior.

Continuity and Change in Adaptation

Demonstrating coherence in individual development does not rest on continuity alone. Change may be comprehended as well. In a current research project (with Byron Egeland, Amos Deinard, and Brain Vaughn) we are following a large sample of poor children from birth to 4½ years. In contrast with our middle-class samples, these children experience noticeably fluctuating environmental circumstances, with life situations changing markedly both toward and away from stability. There are changes in residency, parents' job status, health, substitute care, parents' drug dependency, and perhaps most important, living group membership. People move out and they move in. Separations are common.

These fluctuating circumstances appear linked to the child's quality of adaptation. There is still significant stability in this sample, but there is considerable change, too. For example, whereas 48 of 50 (96 percent) middle-class infants had the same attachment classifications at 12 and 18 months, only 62 of 100 poor children were classified similarly. Most important, changes in the quality of attachment were related to changing life events. Mothers of infants changing from an insecure (Groups A and C) to a secure (Group B) attachment relationship reported a significantly greater reduction in stressful life events than did mothers of infants changing in the other direction (Vaughan et al. 1979). These life-event-related changes provide clear evidence that the individual differences we assess are not simply differences in temperament or socioemotional *g*. Even though changing, the development of these infants is coherent, their pattern of adaptation comprehensible. Nor do these findings suggest that all continuity resides in the environment. All children are vulnerable to stress, but further research may show that some children are more stress resistant and better able to rebound following periods of stress. This would be consistent with a view of the child as an active participant in his or her own development.

Conclusion

There is reason to doubt that children are infinitely resilient, even given the flexibility of our species. Our biology may not be able to adapt to any and all changes in societal conditions proceeding at any rate. What children experience, early and later, makes a difference. We cannot assume that early experiences will somehow be canceled out by later experience. Lasting consequences of early inadequate experience may be subtle and complex, taking the form of increased vulnerability to certain kinds of stress, for example, or becoming manifest only when the individual attempts to establish intimate adult relationships or engage in parenting. But there will be consequences.

To be sure, children have inborn differences in certain behavior characteristics. These characteristics probably influence how we behave toward them (as should be the case if our care is sensitive and responsive). But we shape the persons they are. It is their birthright that the environment to which they must adapt is one that promotes healthy psychological development. It is our obligation to understand the nature of that development.

PART II

Prenatal and Perinatal Influences

The six articles in this section highlight prenatal and perinatal influences on infant development. The first three are concerned with three distinct teratogenic agents—cigarette smoking, alcohol consumption, and obstetrical medication. The remaining three deal with the frequently discussed topics of early mother-infant bonding, the premature infant, and the sudden infant death syndrome.

Landesman-Dwyer and Emmanuel summarize the results of hundreds of studies of the effects of smoking on pregnancy and fetal outcome. The conclusions they reach on the basis of all this work can only be described as sobering: "While all proposed types of damage to the fetus by maternal smoking are not established, one must conclude that smoking is harmful to fetal development. Furthermore, the harmful effects appear to be long-lasting." Indeed, not only does smoking appear to affect fetal growth negatively, but postnatal functional behaviors in the organism are also impaired, leading to lower learning ability in infancy, poorer eventual reading skill, and hyperactivity. Importantly, these detrimental effects are found to be dose related, so that reductions in smoking should occasion concomitant reductions in the risk status of the infant. Unfortunately, while cigarette smoking is the most important single preventable determinant of low birth weight in the United States, smoking by women of childbearing age is more prevalent than ever before. And one can only be depressed by the fact that efforts to date to decrease smoking during pregnancy have not been encouraging.

One observation which Landerman-Dwyer and Emmanuel make regarding smoking is that its detrimental effects on infant development, both prenatally and postnatally, can be heightened when smoking occurs with other problematic behavior, most notably alcohol consumption. Ann Streissguth observes in her article that even without a history of smoking, maternal drinking during pregnancy can have devastating consequences for the infant, including deformity of the facial features and intellectual impairment. Unlike smoking, however, alcohol seems to influence fetal and infant development only when imbibed in great quantities. In the future, after more research has been carried out on babies born to moderate or social drinkers, this conclusion may need to be amended if teratogenic effects can be shown even when alcohol consumption is modest. In the meantime, given the data currently available, it only makes sense for pregnant women to limit their drinking as much as possible, since the integrity of their offspring appears to be at stake.

While smoking and drinking are under the control of mothers themselves, Yvonne Brackbill is concerned with a teratogenic agent that is primarily under the control of others—i.e., obstetricians. In her article, originally a speech delivered to a special congressional committee, Brackbill summarizes the available evidence on the dire effects of obstetrical medication, explains why these effects occur, and raises policy implications for the legislators she was addressing.

As with smoking, the negative effects of obstetrical medication on infant functioning are dose related, and appear to be long-lasting. In the first year, motor skills are most likely to be compromised, and at older ages the capacity to persist at difficult tasks seems to be undermined. The cause of such effects appear to reside in the newborn's limited physiological capabilities, since the neonate, unlike the delivering mother, does not have the biological capability to break down the obstetrical medication biochemically and successfully eliminate it from its system. Thus, these dangerous drugs remain within the infant's system beyond the perinatal period and continue to influence behavior. For Brackbill, the implications of the available evidence are clear: more federally controlled testing of obstetrical medication is required and mothers must be provided with more information regarding the effects of these drugs so they can participate more responsibly in the decision making that determines their use.

Such a pro-maternal orientation is evident in the pioneering work that two physicians, Marshall Klaus and John Kennel, report in the fourth article of this section. Klaus and Kennell have been innovators in the field of postpartum maternity care by providing mothers with opportunities to hold and caress their newborns in the period immediately following parturition. In their paper, Klaus and Kennel summarize the results of several studies that they and their colleagues conducted which tend to indicate that early opportunities for mother-infant bonding can enhance the quality of the developing parent-child relationship.

It is the editor's opinion that the claims of these investigators are exaggerated. And, in support of this position, there exist several recent, carefully controlled investigations, carried out by researchers not ideologically committed to the bonding phenomenon, that fail to replicate the findings reported by Klaus and Kennel. One might rightfully ask, then, why the reading on bonding has been selected for inclusion in this volume. There are two reasons. The first is that Klaus and Kennell's work is provocative and has focused much attention upon the attachment of mothers to their infants, thereby righting an imbalance in the scientific literature which in this area, has focused almost exclusively on the infant's attachment to its caregiver (see the articles by Sroufe [3], Ainsworth [14], and Matas et al. [15] in this volume).

The second and more important reason for including the work on bonding has to do with the dramatic impact that Klaus and Kennell have had on modern maternity care. More than any other persons, these two sensitivie physicians have succeeded in returning the birth process to the family. On the basis of their work, hospitals around the country have altered traditional obstetrical practices and created more humane contexts for childbearing. While the birth process is still treated in many places as an illness, Klaus and Kennell have most certainly initiated what can only be described as a revolution in obstetrical care, one that is working to alter this perception so that pregnancy, labor, and delivery can be treated as normative biological processes from which the family need not be excluded.

It is of interest to note that much of the impetus for Klaus and Kennell's work on mother-newborn contact derived from earlier work on premature and low birth weight infants who, having to be cared for in the hospital, were separated from their mothers for extended periods of time. Data indicating that such at-risk infants were disproportionately likely to be mistreated by their caregivers led Klaus and Kennell to propose that early separation of mother and newborn may impair the development of the early parent-child relationship as it does in several other species of mammals (e.g., sheep, goats). While this suggestion is provocative, the fifth reading in this section alerts us to another explanation.

In her article on prematurity, Susan Goldberg reviews evidence on the developing relationships between mothers and their at-risk infants.

The most notable conclusion she draws from this review is that mothers of premature babies have to "work harder" than mothers of nonrisk infants in maintaining interaction with their offspring. The reason why these mothers "carry more of the interactive burden" is probably because their infants, at least initially, spend less time in alert states and are generally less responsive than full-term infants.

Interestingly, the differences between these two groups of parent-infant dyads tend to disappear toward the end of the first year of life, leading some to suggest that the premature infant elicits from his caregiver a very successful early intervention program. That is, this initially less alert and less responsive child requires from his caregiver greater effort in initiating and maintaining interaction. This eventually pays off by enabling the child to develop, by the last quarter of his first year, the skills possessed by his full-term counterpart, for by this time his interactive engagements with his mother look no different than those of full-term babies, despite their marked early differences.

The fact that prematurity tends to be associated with developmental delay only when coupled with rearing in an at-risk, or economically disadvantaged, environment suggests that under certain conditions these self-initiated intervention processes do not successfully function. Undoubtedly, this is because the caregiver, who is herself under great stress, cannot mobilize the energies to carry the interactive burden that is required when caring for a less responsive organism. Prematurity, then, does not seem to exert an inevitable influence upon infant functioning but rather an influence that is mediated by the context in which the child is reared. In families in which supportive care is provided, premature babies grow up to be indistinguishable from their full-term counterparts. Under impoverished circumstances, however, the "dual risk" of biological and environmental deprivation interact so that the premature infant's development is delayed and sometimes even handicapped.

In the last article in this section, Lewis Lipsitt considers a deprivation more serious than prematurity—the Sudden Infant Death Syndrome (SIDS). As he notes, SIDS is the most common cause of death in the first year of life, excluding the especially hazardous first few post partum days, and accounts for about 10,000 infant deaths each year in the United States. The actual cause of the disturbance remains unknown, but, as Lipsitt points out, progress is being made in understanding its etiology by comparing the birth histories of infants who succumb to crib death and normal control babies. Available evidence suggests that low Apgar scores, histories of perinatal respiratory problems, and minor respiratory disturbances around the time of death (e.g., a cold) are often found in the developmental backgrounds of SIDS victims.

In addition to considering such perinatal and psychophysiological precursors of crib death, Lipsitt offers the provocative hypothesis that infants who succumb to SIDS may be relatively unskilled in protecting themselves from threats to successful respiration and therefore suffocate. Most intriguing is Lipsitt's contention that this inability to protect oneself by, for example, coughing or sneezing to clear respiratory tracks clogged with mucus, may itself represent a learning disability. While involuntary reflex responses protect the organism from threat of occlusion in the first months of life, these are replaced by voluntary acts which are most probably learned between the second and fifth month of life—the time when most crib deaths occur. Thus, the possibility exists that certain infants die because they have a history that places them at risk and then do not acquire those defensive skills necessary to keep their air passages open once involuntary reflex responses disappear.

4

Smoking During Pregnancy

SHARON LANDESMAN-DWYER AND
IRVIN EMANUEL

Scientific studies of the effects of cigarette smoking on the fetus were preceded by warnings based on clinical impressions (Campbell 1936; Bernhard 1948). Sontag and Wallace (1935) showed that fetal heart rate increased with maternal smoking. In laboratory animals, maternal exposure to tobacco smoke led to increased stillbirth and reduced birth weight of offspring (Essenberg, Schwind, & Peters 1940; Schoeneck 1941). Simpson (1957) was the first to demonstrate a birth weight maternal smoking relationship in humans. Soon after, Lowe (1959) published a more comprehensive analysis which dealt with many potential confounding variables, including maternal age, parity, prepregnant weight, and gestational duration. This excellent study confirmed a birth weight effect that survived all attempts at statistical adjustment, as well as a dose response curve also reported by Simpson, and showed that early cessation of smoking minimized harmful effects to the fetus. While the series was small ($N = 2{,}042$), there were suggestions of other effects of smoking, such as increased rates of perinatal mortality, reduced toxemia in pregnancy, and fewer surgical deliveries.

Fetal Growth and Development

The early findings of Simpson and Lowe now are substantially confirmed. In this paper, we are selectively reviewing from 230 articles. More than 45 studies with sample sizes greater than 300 births relate maternal smoking to some problem of reproductive outcome. There now seems to be no question that maternal smoking substantially reduces the birth weight of offspring. This reduction averages about 170–200 gm (Meredith 1975), but ranges from 120 gm to 430 gm, with the largest differences occurring in carefully matched samples (Mulcahy, Murphy, & Martin 1970). There is a significant dose-response relationship and early cessation of smoking can result in birth weights similar to those among offspring of nonsmoking mothers (Frazier et al. 1961; Butler & Alberman 1969; Cope, Lancaster, & Stevens 1973; Murphy & Mulcahy 1971).

The largest studies document an increase in perinatal or neonatal mortality (Butler & Alberman 1969; Andrews & McGarry 1972; Goujard, Rumeau, & Schwartz 1975; Meyer, Jonas, & Tonascia 1976), attributed most often to abruptio placenta, placenta previae, prematurity, pneumonia, and respiratory distress syndrome (Underwood et al. 1967; Comstock et al 1971; Andrews & McGarry, 1972; Goujard, Rumeau, & Schwartz 1975; Meyer, Jonas, & Tonascia 1976; Naeye, Harkness, & Otts 1977). The relative increase in perinatal mortality among smokers' offspring usually is 30–35 percent, although in some studies the risk is more than doubled (Frazier et al. 1961; Comstock et al. 1971; Kaminski, Rumpao, & Schwartz 1978). Some studies report an excess risk for spontaneous abortion in smoking mothers (Zabriskie 1963; Palmgren, Wahlen, & Wallander 1973; Kline, Stein, & Susser 1977), with no indication of increased incidence of abnormal karyotypes (Alberman, Creasy, & Spicer 1976). Sudden infant death syndrome also appears related to smoking during pregnancy (Niswander & Gordon 1972; Naeye, Ladis, & Drage 1976; Rhead 1977).

Besides decreased birth weight, there is a decrease in other anthropometric measures. Shorter birth length is observed in babies of smoking mothers, most markedly among those with poor pregnancy weight gain (Miller et al. 1976). Decreased head circumference also is noted sometimes (Davies et al. 1976; Mau (1976). Deficiency of growth of stature is found in follow-up studies at 6½ years for Canadian children (Dunn et al. 1976) and 11 years for British children (Butler & Goldstein 1973).

There are conflicting data on congenital malformations. It is difficult to resolve these variable findings. Overall, however, cigarette smoking does not appear to be a major factor in congenital malformations.

Significant but small decreases in mean gestational duration, usually one to two days, appear related to smoking (Lowe 1959; Butler & Alberman 1969; Buncher 1969). Some studies, again those with smaller sample sizes, are not in agreement (Bailey 1970; Kullander & Källen 1971; Desouza, John, & Richards 1976). In addition, increases in the percentage of preterm gestations frequently are detected (Herriot, Bollewicz, & Hythens 1962; Reinke & Henderson 1966; Andrews & McGarry 1972; Meyer Jonas, & Tonascia 1976).

Behavioral Effects

The most important recent findings focus on the functional consequences of maternal smoking on offspring. Within minutes of maternal smoking, decreased breathing movements and increased heart rate can be detected in the fetus (Sontag & Wallace 1935; Hellman et al. 1961) lasting an average of 90 minutes (Manning & Feyerabend 1976). From carefully controlled experiments, it is clear that these immediate effects of maternal smoking are linked most closely to nicotine content, rather than to carbon monoxide or to other components of cigarette smoke (Gennser, Marsal, & Brantmark 1975; Manning & Feyerabend 1976). A significant dose-response curve is demonstrated for apnea and for decreased fetal breathing movements, with the greatest effects observed in fetuses who ultimately are small-for-dates at birth (Manning & Feyerabend 1976).

With one exception (O'Lane 1963), significant differences in newborns' Apgar scores are not found (Peterson, Morese, & Kaltreida 1965; Russell, Taylor, & Law 1968; Kullander & Kallen 1971; Cope, Lancaster & Stevens 1973). A prospective study, utilizing detailed behavioral assessment techniques, reports significant interaction effects for maternal smoking and moderate to heavy alcohol consumption. Martin et al. (1977) find that neonates exposed prenatally to greater amounts of both nicotine (estimated by amount and brand smoked) and alcohol (average daily amount of absolute alcohol) perform significantly worse on two operant conditioning tasks—head turning and sucking. Landesman-Dwyer, Keller, & Streissguth (1978) observe that offspring of heavier smoking and drinking women display significantly more coughing and sneezing, increased atypical head orientation to the left, and decreased alert visual behavior. The predictive significance of these neonatal behavioral findings for subsequent development is not yet known.

Long-term behavioral effects of maternal smoking have emerged in three major studies: (1) the British National Child Development Study of more than 12,000 children studied from birth to 11 years of age (Davie, Butler, & Goldstein, 1972; Butler & Goldstein 1973); (2) a Canadian study of 319 children evaluated from birth to 6½ years (Dunn et al. 1977); and (3) the Collaboratove Perinatal Project that followed more than 28,000 American children from birth to 7 years of age (Nichols, 1977).

Davie, Butler, & Goldstein (1972) report significant decrements in reading ability and social adjustment in 7 years olds. For the 11-year-olds, Butler and Goldstein (1973) find that smokers' offspring are significantly lower in general ability, reading comprehension, and mathematics skills than are offspring of nonsmokers, even after adjusting for social class, maternal age, maternal height, sex of child and number of older and younger siblings. These decrements in performance, however, are not as large as those attributable to social class or to number of older and younger siblings.

The results of Dunn et al. (1977) are similar, showing that cognitive abilities, as measured on eight standardized tests, are compromised by Caucasian children whose mothers smoked during pregnancy. Grade placement, IQ, perceptual motor abilities, and linguistic skills are significantly lower in the offspring of smokers. In addition, "minimal cerebral dysfunction" is diagnosed by physicians nearly twice as frequently in smokers' children, and male offspring of smokers are rated by teachers as significantly more misbehaved in school than are controls. Social class, which differs significantly between smokers and nonsmokers (Dunn et al. 1976), is controlled for in the analysis of IQ scores, but not the other outcome measures.

Additional confirmation comes from Nichols (1977), who reports a significant relationship between maternal smoking during pregnancy and behavior in seven-year-olds. Specifically, amount of cigarettes smoked during pregnancy relates significantly to increased hyperactivity, low achievement, and soft neurological signs in offspring.

Animals exposed to nicotine prenatally are significantly more active than controls (Martin & Becker 1970). One retrospective study in humans notes that hyperactive children are significantly more likely to have mothers who smoked more during pregnancy than are normal or nonhyperactive dyslexic children (Denson, Nanson, & McWatters 1975). Although hyperactivity has been associated with increased minor physical anomalies (Waldrop et al. 1978), these have not been assessed carefully in offspring of smokers.

Modes of Action

Because cigarette smoke is chemically complex, there are many possibilities for the modes of action (i.e., processes of influence) which are not definitely established. Hypothesized modes of action for the birth weight reduction include:

1. Action of nicotine on uterine vessels (Manning & Feyerabend 1976);
2. Direct action of nicotine on the fetus (Sontag & Wallace 1935), which may result in accelerated fetal metabolism and greater need for nuturients;
3. Reduced maternal weight gain (Andrews & McGarry 1972; Naeye, Harkness, & Otts 1977). To date, however, other studies fail to substantiate a reduction of maternal weight gain (Jarvinen & Osterlund 1963; Mau 1976);
4. Decreased availability of important nutrients, e.g., amino acids and zinc, possibly related to detoxification of cyanide;
5. Chronic fetal hypoxia associated with increased levels of carboxyhemoglobin (Haddon, Nesbitt, & Garcia 1961; Astrup et al. 1972; Spira et al. 1975; Longo 1976);

6. Enzyme poisoning by carbon monoxide (Mantell 1964); and
7. Decreased immune response associated with increased maternal urinary tract and viral infections (Nymand 1974). All these hypothetical possibilities deserve further study.

Conclusions

While all proposed types of damage to the fetus by maternal smoking are not established, one must conclude that smoking is harmful to fetal development. Furthermore, the harmful effects appear to be long-lasting. As pointed out by Garn et al. (1977), smoking is the most important single preventable determinant of low birth weight in the United States. Unfortunately, smoking in women of childbearing age is more prevalent than ever, and attempts to influence smoking during pregnancy have not had results and have not been encouraging or strongly endorsed by medical practitioners (Jones 1975; Graham 1976; Donovan 1977).

Even though the nicotine and tar content of cigarettes has decreased, there does not seem to be a significant beneficial effect on birth weight or perinatal mortality (Newcombe 1976). Also, filtered cigarettes do not reduce the birth weight deficit (Underwood et al. 1967). Based on information available, prevention of the harmful effects of tobacco on the fetus can come only from cessation of smoking.

5

Maternal Alcoholism and the Outcome of Pregnancy

A Review of the Fetal Alcohol Syndrome

ANN PYTKOWICZ STREISSGUTH

Alcohol and pregnancy have a long history of incompatibility that has been all but ignored in modern times. Despite age-old warnings, there has been virtually no systematic research on the effects of alcohol on the fetus until the past decade. This paper will describe in detail the Seattle research which culminated in identifiying the "fetal alcohol syndrome," and will discuss the present body of literature pertaining to the fetal alcohol syndrome.

Growth Deficiency and Development Delay

In 1969, Christy Ulleland, a young pediatric resident at Harborview Medical Center in Seattle, became interested in infants who failed to thrive despite the best medical care that could be provided. This bothered Ulleland, and she looked more carefully into their backgrounds. She made the astute observation that one environmental factor shared by these infants was that they had alcoholic mothers. The significance of failure to thrive in infants of alcoholic mothers is important because of the suspicion of poor care that is implicitly assumed, perhaps unjustly, when the history of maternal alcoholism is revealed. The fact that these children continued to fail to thrive when given proper care suggested to Ulleland that the prenatal impact of the mothers' alcoholism might be of more importance in their growth deficiency than the type of care the mothers had provided after delivery.

Ulleland examined the records of all infants born at the Harborview during an eight-month period. She looked for infants who were undergrown for gestational age, were hospitalized for failure to thrive, or had alcoholic mothers. From the total of 1,582 records she identified 12 alcoholic mothers. The proportion of undergrown babies (below the 10th percentile) born to these alcoholic mothers was 83 percent; the proportion of undergrown babies among the nonalcoholic mothers was 2.3 percent. The hospital serves primarily a low socioeconomic urban population. Detailed nutritional histories retrospectively obtained from seven of the alocholic mothers revealed several whose diets had been deficient during pregnancy, including two with diets that were severely deficient in calories and protein.

Ten of the twelve babies born to alcoholic mothers were given developmental tests: two were normal, three borderline, and five retarded. Clearly, this study points out the high risks to the infants of alcoholic women.

Identification of the Fetal Alcohol Syndrome

In early 1973, while attending a pediatric clinic at Harborview, David W. Smith (a dysmorphologist) saw one of the children whom Ulleland had identified and was struck by the lad's unusual facies, particularly the small palpebral fissures. He felt sure the child had a syndrome but did not recognize it as one that was labeled. Because the mother was an alcoholic, Smith asked to see others of Ulleland's group of children of alcoholic mothers. Eight of the original patients were brought into the clinic on the same day for Smith and Kenneth Jones (a dysmorphology fellow) to examine. When the physicians lined up the children and looked at them as a group, it was obvious that four of the eight had the same condition. Smith and Jones then went through their own files of unidentified, unusual looking children to see if any had clear histories of maternal alcoholism. Three such cases were identified, and these children were brought to the clinic. They too had the same characteristics as the original four examined. Smith and Jones were then quite certain that they had "uncovered" a link between maternal alcoholism and dysmorphogenesis in offspring of female alcoholics.

The very next week Smith was invited to give a visiting lectureship at Akron, Ohio, and was asked the type of patients that he wanted to see while in Akron. Smith requested any child of an alcoholic mother. When he described the expected features of such a child, the resident making the arrangements said that he had just seen such a patient and would make the child available. When Smith was presented the child at grand rounds, the characteristic features were clearly present.

The pattern of altered growth and morphogenesis described in these first eight clinical cases, all born to chronic alcoholic mothers, included the following:

1. Prenatal growth deficiency characterized by short birth length and low birth weight. Although the mean gestational age was 38 weeks, the mean birth length and birth weight were at the 50th percentile for gestational ages of 34 and 33 weeks, respectively.
2. Postnatal growth deficiency characterized by continuing failure to thrive. At age 1 these children's growth rate was only 65 percent of normal for length and 38 percent of normal for weight.
3. Craniofacial abnormalities, including microcephaly, short palpebral fissures, maxillary hypoplasia, and epicanthal folds.
4. Joint and limb anomalies, including altered palmar crease pattern.
5. Cardiac defects, primarily septal defects.
6. Mental deficiency. The mean IQ on standardized intelligence tests was 67, with a range from 83 to below 50.
7. Delayed motor development, both gross and fine motor, including tremulousness, weak grasp, and poor eye-hand coordination.

Mothers and foster mothers of these children reported that the children had often been hard to feed (especially as infants), had not nursed well, often had a poor suck, and were generally disinterested in food. A high proportion of the children were reported to have engaged in repetitive self-stimulating behaviors such as head banging, head rolling, and rocking.

Confirmation in a Nonclinical Sample

In June 1974, Jones, Smith, Streissguth, and Myrianthopoulos published a study that was not a clinical study. In this they used data from the Collaborative Perinatal Project of the National Institute of Neurologic Disease and Stroke, a national propsective study of 55,000 pregnancies in which the offspring were followed up to 7 years of age. Although the women had not been systematically questioned regarding their alcoholism histories or drinking habits, 69 subjects had been classified as alcoholic on their medical records. After perusal of these records, a sample of 23 subjects was drawn in which the history of alcoholism during pregnancy was clearly substantiated. Two nonalcoholic control women were matched to each of the 23 alcoholic mothers, matching on the basis of socioeconomic status, education, age, race, parity, marital status, and geographic region of residence.

The findings in this well-controlled study, in which all the data were gathered blind, are sobering. Four of the offspring of the alcoholic mothers died within the first week of life, a perinatal mortality of 17 percent, compared to 2 percent in the controls. Six of the nineteen surviving children born to alcoholic mothers had enough abnormal features to suggest the possibility of fetal alcohol syndrome on the basis of the physical findings alone; none of the controls were so affected. Thus a total of 43 percent of the offspring of the alcoholic mothers either died or appeared to have had fetal alcohol syndrome as compared to 2 percent of the matched controls (presumably nonalcoholic).

Forty-four percent of the surviving offspring of alcoholic women in this study had borderline to moderate mental deficiency (IQ 79 or below at age 7 years) compared to 9 percent of the controls.

As table 5.1 indicates, children of chronically alcoholic mothers had significantly lower intelligence at 7 years of age when compared to carefully matched controls. As the table also indicates, at age 7 this sample of children born to alcoholic mothers had significant retardation in all three areas of academic achievement compared to their carefully matched controls.

Several related findings from this study are worthy of note: although group differences in mean IQ scores were highly significant at age 7, nevertheless, 2 of the 15 children of the chronically alcoholic women had IQ scores between 100 and 109. Thus it is clear that not all children born to these alcoholic mothers were uniformly impaired.

The striking differences in intelligence were not demonstrated until the children were older; earlier assessments during infancy and preschool years had not shown such marked discrepancy between groups. This finding could mean that the extent of the prenatal insult sustained by the children of alcoholic mothers was not fully apparent until they were at an age when higher level cognitive functioning was measurable. Or, on the other hand, it could reflect real differences in the postnatal environ-

Table 5.1 Performance of Offspring of Alcoholic Mothers Compared to Matched Controls (Mean Scores)

	Offspring of Alcoholic Mothers	Offspring of Matched Controls	t	p
WISC[1] Full Scale IQ	81	95	−2.85	0.007
WISC Verbal IQ	82	92	−1.96	0.035
WISC Performance IQ	82	99	−3.05	0.005
WRAT[2] Spelling	79	94	−2.20	0.023
WRAT Reading	86	95	−1.79	0.048
WRAT Arithmetic	84	94	−2.34	0.018

NOTE: n = 15 offspring of alcoholic mothers and 30 matched controls, all tested at age 7. (Scores reported are all standard scores, where $\bar{X}$ = 100 and the standard deviation = 15).

[1] Wechsler Intelligence Scale for Children

[2] Wide Range Achievement Test

ments of the two groups of children or an interaction effect between prenatal and postnatal environments.

Less than half of the children of alcoholic mothers in this study were still living with their natural mothers by age 7, compared to over 90 percent of the controls. Children remaining with their alcoholic mothers tended to have a lower intelligence at age 7, although this difference was not statistically significant.

Conclusions

The fetal alcohol syndrome is a recently recognized pattern of growth deficiency, altered morphogenesis, and mental deficiency that occurs in some children whose mothers were chronically alcoholic and drinking heavily during pregnancy. The characteristic facies, particularly the small eyes and flattened nasal bridge, make the syndrome easily recognizable at birth as well as during childhood. Diagnosis, especially in children having learning and adaptational problems, is important because it clarifies the primary etiology and provides the opportunity for recommending against subsequent pregnancies for alcoholic women who continue to drink heavily.

Even in the absence of the physical manifestations of the fetal alcohol syndrome, it is clear that children whose mothers were chronically alcoholic during pregnancy may be at risk for a variety of learning and behavioral handicaps that are only recently being recognized. We can only begin to speculate at the degree to which the hyperactivity, poor attention spans, poor eye-hand coordination, slightly delayed development, and mild learning problems of children might represent the effects of maternal alcoholism.

Studies to date have only been of chronically alcoholic mothers, primarily of the lower social classes. To what extent the offspring of moderate or heavy social drinkers may be a risk is not clear because the prospective studies are still in the data-gathering stage.

Many questions remain unanswered: What is the level of alcohol necessary to compromise the fetus? What are the compounding effects of alcohol with other drugs? What are the individual differences in mothers and fetuses that may make some fetuses more vulnerable to insult? What are the other variables related to the degree of functional disability experienced by the child? Much research is needed, including many more clinical studies of families of alcoholic mothers studied longitudinally. However, the risk of damage to the fetus is clear in chronically alcoholic women who continue to drink heavily during pregnancy.

6

Lasting Behavioral Effects of Obstetric Medication on Children

Research Findings and Public Policy Implications

YVONNE BRACKBILL

This article will discuss the lasting behavioral effects of obstetric medication on infants and children—a research area in which I have been involved for the past decade.

Back in the 1960s, one of my graduate students told me that she wanted to do a thesis on the effects on infant behavior of obstetric medication, i.e., the anesthetics and analgesics given mothers during labor and delivery. (By behavior, I mean the ability to see and hear, the development of motor skills, language ability, intelligence, and so on.) She explained that she had been bothered by the possibility that her second child might have sustained brain damage from obstetric medication, and that she was motivated by her lingering anger at having been given such medication against her will. I told her I thought the question would already have been thoroughly researched by obstetricians since they had been using anesthesia for delivery for a century and since the question of possible damage was such an obvious one. The graduate student proved me wrong: there was no body of literature on the subject.

The study that she and I conducted was the beginning of systematic research on the effects of obstetric medication on infant behavior. At present there are some 35 studies on that topic. The investigators are a diverse lot, and the laboratories are scattered throughout the United States and Great Britain. Nevertheless, the major findings, summarized below, are clear, consistent and unequivocal.

The basis for the problem is that the human baby's anatomical and physiological development is not complete at the time it is born. There are two very important ways in which the newborn is immature. One concerns the central nervous system. Important areas of the brain are still undeveloped at birth. The production and development of neural elements probably continues in the cerebellum for 1.5 years and in the hippocampus for 4.5 years. During this period of rapid brain growth, the brain is especially vulnerable to damage. Also, it is especially easy for toxins to reach the brain in neonates because the so-called "barrier" between blood and brain is immature as well. The second important way in which the newborn infant is immature is that the liver and kidneys—the organs most needed for drug metabolism and excretion—are not fully functional at time of birth.

So, then, the situation is this: the newborn human being is an organism poorly positioned for dealing with drugs. They lodge in brain structures that are still developing and are therefore at high risk to damage. They are not readily transformed to non-toxic compounds since the necessary liver functions are immature. And they are not readily excreted because of inefficient kidney function.

From all these considerations, it would be small wonder if obstetrical medication agents did *not* inflict some mischief on the infant.

What are the behavioral effects of obstetric medication and how have they been studied? The 35 investigations I have mentioned have studied healthy, full-term babies who came from low risk pregnancies and whose deliveries were normal and uneventful. (In this way one avoids confusing the effects of drugs with the effects of pre-existing disease or complications.) Most of the studies were done on newborns, though a few included older babies. The most important study is the National Institutes of Health's Collaborative Perinatal Project, a longitudinal study of over 50,000 children which Congress authorized in the 1950s. Dr. Sally Broman and I have finished analyzing the results of this study for 3,500 of its most healthy babies tested at four months, eight months, and twelve months. We are now analyzing obstetric medication for the same children tested at four years and seven years.

Looking at the results of all 35 studies, almost all have found statistically significant behavioral effects of obstetric medication. Furthermore, the direction of these effects is uniformly, without exception, toward behavioral degradation and interference with normal function. *No* study has ever demonstrated or even suggested that obstetric medication improves normal functioning.

A second general finding is that obstetric medication effects are more pronounced in some behavioral areas than others. During the first year of life, the strongest effects can be seen in the development of gross motor abilities—e.g., limitations in the ability to sit, to stand, and to locomote. They can also be seen in certain emerging cognitive functions, principally the development of inhibitory ability—e.g., the ability to *stop* responding to redundant signals, to *stop* crying when comforted, to *stop* responding to distracting stimuli. During later years, the strongest effects can be seen in the development of language and associated cognitive skills. At all ages, the effects are more clearly visible when tasks are difficult, i.e., when they require the child to exert itself, to make an effort, to cope with problems.

A third general finding is that the behavioral effects of obstetric medication are dose related and potency related. That is, stronger drugs and larger doses of a single drug produce stronger behavioral effects. For example, general anesthetics have stronger effects than local anesthetics, and local anesthetics have stronger effects than no anesthetic at all.

The most important general finding is that the behavioral effects of obstetric medication are not transient. They persist. Within the age range for which we have data—one day to seven years—there is some evidence of decrease for a few drugs. But for the other drugs, most notably inhalant anesthetics, the adverse effects are as strong at four years as they are at one year. It is difficult to avoid concluding that the damage is permanent.

Now I will turn to three issues that help pull these empirical data into the perspective of health policy and planning.

The first of these issues is the increase over the years in obstetric drug administration. There seems to be a widespread misconception among the medical and nonmedical community alike that the number of drugs administered during labor and delivery is decreasing. This is not true. In point of fact, it is increasing. On the whole, I estimate that 95 percent of births in United States hospitals nowadays are medicated. This means 3,500,000 medicated births out of 3,700,000 total births per year. If the average IQ loss per medicated birth is four points, this means 14,060,000 IQ points lost to new U.S. citizens every year. Cumulatively, that figure should put the problem of obstetric medication at the head of the class of national health priorities.

The second important issue to bring to your attention is the question of accountability in monitoring adverse reactions from these drugs and in controlling their distribution for clinical use. The United States does not monitor these or other adverse drug reactions, as Senator Kennedy has pointed out. Neither does it effectively control the use of drugs commonly used in obstetric medication but never scientifically evaluated for that purpose. The drugs I'm talking about have all been cleared for clinical use by the Federal Drug Administration. However, the research that served as a basis for FDA clearance was carried out on adults. None has been done using infant subjects. Pharmacological tests results from adults cannot automatically be extrapolated to infants because the neonate's response to drugs is often quantitatively different. If we insist on administering drugs to infants, the infant itself must be the object of pharmacological study. Nevertheless, such studies are not carried out by the manufacturers of obstetric drugs nor are they required by the FDA as a precondition for clearing drugs for clinical use.

Who is responsible for this situation? The FDA claims that it is not responsible for policing the uses to which a drug is put.

The drug industry claims that it is not responsible for testing a new drug for all potential uses. From the perspective of child health and welfare, the issue of monitoring and controlling obstetric drugs exists in a vacuum of accountability.

The last policy issue to bring to your attention is a consumer issue: who decides what, if any, drugs a mother will take and how much? The medical community claims that mothers receive medication only when they request it for pain or when there are birth complications. Although there are no data allowing direct evaluation of this claim, there are indirect sources of evidence. Collectively, they indicate that mothers do not receive adequate information on adverse drug reactions, on differences among drug risks, or on alternatives to drugs for relief from pain. They also indicate that women have little voice in deciding which if any drugs they will consume.

For many illnesses today, drug therapy is the only effective therapy. Under these circumstances, there's very little real decision-making involved. But pregnancy is not an illness. Childbirth is not an illness. Administering drugs prenatally and perinatally is more often optional than essential, and there is plenty of room for decision making.

One additional point about the mother as decision maker. In a very real way, the physician protects himself/herself by allowing the mother to share in the decision making process: When the mother takes more responsibility for decision making, the physician takes less responsibility and to that extent makes himself/herself less vulnerable to charges of malpractice.

7

Parent-to-Infant Attachment

MARSHALL H. KLAUS AND
JOHN H. KENNELL

The impetus to study the mother-to-infant bond intensively occurred 10 to 15 years ago when staffs of intensive care nurseries observed that sometimes, after all extraordinary efforts had been taken to save small premature infants, they would return to emergency rooms battered and partially destroyed by their parents even though they had been sent home intact and thriving. More careful studies of this phenomenon have consistently shown that battering and failure-to-thrive without organic cause appear in a disproportionate number of infants who were premature or hospitalized for other reasons during the newborn period. Re-analysis of a number of these studies has shown an association between early separation and these disastrous conditions.

Over the last six years, however, more and more mothers have been allowed to enter premature nurseries in the United States. Nonetheless, in a recent survey of 1,400 nurseries in the United States done in 1970 by Barnett and Grobstein (1974), only 30 percent of mothers were permitted to enter nurseries and of these, only 40 percent allowed the mother to touch her baby in the first days of life. It is apparent from the data and definition of deprivation (Barnett et al. 1970) that most normal deliveries in the United States are followed by several days of deprivation for the mother. A woman who delivers a premature infant suffers complete deprivation from the first day if she can only see her infant through a glass window for eight weeks. Only mothers who deliver at home and room in with their infants from the moment of birth experience no deprivation.

Species-Specific Behavior

Detailed observations of many species have shown that adaptive species-specific patterns of behavior, including nesting, exploring, grooming and retrieving, before, during and after parturition have evolved to meet the needs of the young.

For example, the domestic cat behaves in a characteristic way at the time of delivery. Towards the end of her pregnancy, she finds a warm dark place, preferably with a soft surface, in which to give birth. Throughout labor and delivery, she spends increasingly more time licking her genital region. After delivery, she continues licking, but with the newborn kitten as her object. The placenta is usually promptly eaten. After the birth of the last kitten, the mother lies down encircling her kittens, and rests with them for about 12 hours (Schneirla, Rosenblatt, Tobach 1963). Each mammalian species studied has its own characteristic behavioral sequence around the time of delivery and following the birth (Hersher, Richmond, & Moore 1963).

We have searched for similar specific behavior in the human mother in the hope that close observations of very early interaction between mother and infant might provide clues or principles that may not be evident at other times. If humans exhibit such specific patterns of behavior, knowledge of the sequence might be clinically applicable in situations where mothers and infants are at present separated early, such as prematurity or sickness during the neonatal period. In addition, it is our hypothesis that there is an immediate interlocking, and a reciprocal set of behaviors for attachment which must quickly operate because of the infant's precarious state after delivery.

Filmed observations made after delivery in a hospital show that a mother presented with her nude, full-term infant begins with fingertip touching of the infant's extremities and within a few minutes proceeds to massaging, encompassing palm contact of the trunk (Klaus et al. 1970). Mothers of premature infants in incubators also follow a small portion of this sequence but proceed at a much slower rate.

In sharp contrast to the woman who gives birth in the hospital, a woman delivering at home with a midwife appears to be in control. She chooses both the room in the house and the location within the room where she would like the birth to take place as well as the close friends who will be present to share this experience with her. She is an active participant rather than a passive patient during her labor and delivery. Immediately after delivery, she appears to be in a remarkable state of ecstasy. In fact many mothers have reported they had sensations similar to orgasm at the time of delivery (Lang 1974). The exuberance is contagious and the observers share the festive mood of unreserved elation after the delivery. Striking in films is the observers' intense interest in the infant, especially in the first 15 to 20 minutes of life. Although controlled studies have not yet been done to test the effects of this experience on the mother-infant relationship, it seems clear that the conditions surrounding delivery greatly affect the mother's initial mood and interaction with her infant.

In the observed home deliveries, the mother cradles her infant in her arms immediately after his birth and begins touching his face with her fingertips. Thus, we have fragmentary evidence that human mothers engage in a species-specific sequence of touching behaviors when first meeting their infants even though the speed and pattern of this sequence may be modified by environmental conditions.

A Sensitive Period

It has been found that in a large number of animal species, separation of mother and baby immediately afer birth can severely distort mothering behavior. For example, if the goat is separated for 1 hour from her kid immediately after delivery, she is likely to butt it away when it is returned. However, if a separation of similar duration begins 10 minutes after delivery, the dam will reaccept her kid upon reunion and allow it to nurse (Klopfer 1971). Thus, there appears to be a sensitive period in the first minutes of life in which any alteration in the normal pattern of interaction can result in aberrant subsequent mothering behavior.

There is evidence that when human mothers are separated from their babies during the first hours and days after delivery, they may have difficulty forming an attachment. Studies of mothers of premature infants who spent their first weeks of life in neonatal intensive care nurseries highlight this problem. In those nurseries where the mothers are not allowed to visit, doctors find that mothers temporarily forget they have babies and find reasons to put off taking them home.

A small number of studies have focused on the possibility of an early sensitive period in the human mother. Observations at Stanford and in our own unit have been made with mothers of prematures, half of whom were permitted into the nursery in the first hours and half of whom could not come in until the twentieth day. At Case Western Reserve University, mothers who had early contact with their infants looked at them significantly more than late contact mothers during a filmed feeding at the time of discharge. Furthermore, preliminary data on the IQs of these two groups of children at 42 months indicate that children in the early contact group scored significantly higher (mean = 99) than did children in the late contact group (mean = 85). Strikingly, a significant correlation was found between IQ at 42 months and the amount of time women looked at their babies during the one-month filmed feeding ($r = 0.71$). This is consistent with our hypothesis that early contact affects aspects of maternal behavior which may have significance for the child's later development. At Stanford, when mothers separated from their premature babies from 3 to 12 weeks were compared with those of prematures permitted early contact, there were more divorces (five compared to one) and more infants relinquished (two compared to none) in the group of mothers with prolonged separation

(Leifer et al. 1972). It should be noted that these were all middle-class families and they all had initially planned on keeping their infants.

During the past five years, six studies of the sensitive period of mothers and their full-term infants have either been completed or are underway.

In a tightly controlled study of 28 primiparous mothers and their full-term infants, half the mothers were given 1 hour in the first 3 hours and 15 more hours of contact with their infants in the first three days of life than were the controls. The mothers who had early and extended contact were more likely to stand near their infants and watch during the physical examination, showed significantly more soothing behavior, engaged in more eye-to-eye contact and fondling during feeding, and were more reluctant to leave their infants with someone else at one month than were mothers not given the extended contact experience (Klaus et al. 1972). At one year the two groups of mothers were still significantly different. Extended contact mothers spent more time near the table assisting the physician and soothing their infant while he was being examined, and reported themselves to be more preoccupied with the baby when they went out (Kennell et al. 1974). At two years, when the linguistic behaviors of the two groups of mothers while speaking to their children were compared, extended contact mothers asked twice as many questions, and used more words per proposition, fewer content words, more adjectives, and fewer commands than did the controls (Ringler et al. 1975). It is impressive evidence for a sensitive maternal period that just 16 extra hours of contact in the first three days of life had such far-reaching effects.

In a small but carefully controlled study, Winters (1973) gave six mothers in one group their babies to suckle shortly after birth and compared these with six mothers who did not have contact with their babies until approximately 16 hours later. All had originally intended to breast feed and none stopped because of physical problems. When checked two months later, all six mothers who had suckled their babies on the delivery table were still breast feeding, whereas only one of the other six was still nursing.

Recently, Kennell, Klaus, Mata, Sosa, and Urrutia started a long-term study in two hospitals in Guatemala. In the Social Security Hospital, members of one group of 19 mothers were given their babies on the delivery table during the episiotomy repair period, then allowed to stay with them in privacy for 45 minutes. Each mother-infant pair was nude under a heat panel. Members of the other group of mothers were separated from their babies shortly after delivery, in the routine for both hospitals. Except for this difference in initial contact, the care of the two groups was identical. The infants were discharged with free milk at two days, as is the practice of the hospital.

When the babies were checked at 35 and 90 days after birth, the mean weight of those in the early contact group was significantly greater than that of the control group. The socioeconomic, marital, housing, and income status of the mothers in the two groups were not significantly different.

In Roosevelt Hospital in Guatemala, a similar study was carried out and at 35 days there were no significant differences in weight gain. Other data are not yet available to help account for these discrepant findings.

In Pelotis, Brazil, Sousa et al. (1974) recently compared the success of breast feeding during the first two months of life in two groups of 100 women who delivered normal full-term babies in a 20-bed maternity ward. In the study group, the newborn baby was put to breast immediately after birth and continuous contact between the mother and baby was maintained during the lying-in period. The baby lay in a cot beside his mother's bed. The control group had the traditional contact with their infants—a glimpse shortly after birth and then visits for approximately 30 minutes every 3 hours, starting 12 to 14 hours after birth. The babies were kept in a separate nursery. Successful breast feeding was defined as the mother's not using complementary feedings other than tea, water, or small amounts of fruit juice until two months after birth. At two months of age, 77 percent of the early contact mothers were successfully breast feeding in contrast to only 27 percent of the controls. A weakness in this design which limits the strength of the findings is that during the experimental period there was a special nurse working in the unit to stimulate and encourage breast feeding. Although not definitive in itself, this study adds weight to our hypothesis.

In a third study in 1974 at Roosevelt Hospital in Guatemala, members of a different group, of nine mothers, were given their babies nude under a heat panel after they had left the delivery room. Members of a second group, of 10, were separated according to the usual routine. The babies in both groups were sent to the newborn nursery for the next 12 hours, after which they went to the mother in a seven-bed room for the first breast feeding. At 12 hours, each mother's interactions with her infant were noted by an observer who did not know to which group they belonged. Observations of the mother's fondling, kissing, looking "en face," gazing at, and holding her baby close were made for 15 seconds of every minute for 15 minutes. The group with early contact showed significantly increased attachment behaviors.

Studies of the effects of rooming-in have also confirmed the importance of the early postnatal period. At Duke University a number of years ago, an incrase in breast feeding and a reduction in anxious phone calls was noted when rooming-in was instituted (McBryde 1951). In Sweden, mothers randomly assigned to rooming-in arrangements were more confident and felt more competent in caregiving. They also appeared to be more sensitive to the crying of their own infants than were mothers who did not have the rooming-in experience (Greenberg, Rosenberg, & Lind 1973). In an interesting and significant observation of fathers, Lind (1973) noted that paternal caregiving was markedly increased in the first three months of life when the father was asked to undress the infant twice and establish eye-to-eye contact with him for an hour during the first three days of life.

Practical Considerations

Until 100 years ago, events surrounding the delivery had changed little. Elaborate customs of the society helped parents through this time. In the last century, however, increasing emphasis has been placed on the medical and scientific aspects of delivery but less attention has been paid to the equally valid psychological considerations. A question may be raised: has the enormous improvement in medical management, which has lessened the physical dangers, contributed to a waning concern about the many other problems a mother faces during pregnancy? In 1959, Bibring wrote, "What was once a crisis with carefully worked-out traditional customs of giving support to the woman passing through this crisis-period has become at this time a crisis with no mechanisms within the society for helping the woman involved in this profound change of conflict-solutions and adjustive tasks." This deficiency accounts for the development of the many support systems in our society. The wide assortment of childbirth classes which attempt to continue previous customs are good examples. These groups help the mother through the delivery period as well as aid her in later infant and child care. They also lessen the tensions, fears and fantasies that occur during normal pregnancies. By joining a group of mothers, with whom she can chat and share her feelings, a woman can alleviate the many emotional upsets that occur during normal pregnancy. We therefore believe that these courses, particularly those in which mothers participate actively, have a valuable supportive role during pregnancy.

To minimize the number of unknowns for a mother while she is in the hospital, she and her husband should visit the maternity unit to see where labor and delivery will take place. She should also learn about the anaesthetic (if she is to receive one), delivery routines, and all the procedures and medication she will receive before, during, and after delivery. By reducing the possibility of surprise, such advance preparation will increase confidence during labor and delivery. For an adult, just as for a child entering the hospital for surgery, and more meticulously every step and event is detailed in advance, the less the subsequent anxiety. The less anxiety the mother experiences while delivering and becoming attached to her baby, the better will be her immediate relationship with him.

The mother must have continuing support and reassurance during her labor and delivery, whether from her husband, a midwife, or a nurse. She also must be satisfied with the arrangements that have been made to maintain her home during her hospitalization. In Holland, when the mothers deliver at home, mother-helpers come into the home at the time of delivery and take over the care of the family. The mother-helper helps the midwife to deliver the infant. This gives the mother the freedom to concentrate on the needs of the baby and to enjoy her family in the process, and it relieves pressure on the father, reserving his energies for the family.

In an effort to reduce the amount of tension on the mother, she should labor and deliver in the same room, preventing the necessity of rushing to a delivery room in the last minutes of labor. Once the delivery is completed and the mother has had a quick glance at the infant, it is important for her to have a few seconds to regain her composure and, in a sense, catch her breath before she proceeds to the next task—taking on the infant. This breath-catching usually occurs during the period when the placenta is being delivered, while the mother is being cleansed and is having any necessary suturing. It has been our experience that it is best not to give a mother her baby until she indicates that she is ready to take it on. It should be her decision.

In many hospitals it is customary to put the baby on the mother's chest for 1 or 2 minutes shortly after delivery. This is helpful but, coupled with the lack of privacy, the narrow table and the short time period, it does not allow sufficient opportunity for the mother to touch and explore her baby. Although it is a reasonable procedure, it is not sufficient to optimize maternal attachment.

After delivery, it is extremely valuable for the father, mother, and baby to have a period alone in either the delivery room or an adjacent room (i.e., a recovery room). Obviously, this is only possible if the infant is normal and the mother is well. The mother should have the infant with her on the bed so she can hold him. The infant should not be off in a bassinet where she can only see his face. She should be given the baby nude and allowed to examine him completely. We have found it valuable to encourage the mother to move over in her regular hospital bed, so that she only takes up about half of it, leaving the other half for her partially dressed or nude infant. A heat panel easily maintains or, if need be, increases the body temperature of the infant.

Several mothers have told us of the unforgettable experience of holding their nude baby against their own bare chest, so we recommended skin-to-skin contact. The father sits or stands at the side of the bed by the infant. This allows the parents and infant to become acquainted. Because the eyes are so important for both the parents and baby, we withold the application of silver nitrate to the eys until after this rendezvous.

We have found it valuable for the mother, father, and infant to be together for about 30 minutes. After 10 to 15 minutes, the mother and baby often fall into a deep sleep. In Guatemalan hospitals, where drugs and anaesthesia are used more sparingly, most mothers were usually awake after 45 minutes of privacy with their infants. The mother and father never forget this significant and stimulating shared experience. It helps to firmly bond the actual, real infant to both parents. We must emphasize that this should be a private session.

Affectional bonds are further consolidated in the succeeding four to five days through continued close association of baby and mother, particularly when she cares for him. Close contact with her husband and other children is also obviously important.

8

Prematurity

Effects on Parent-Infant Interaction

SUSAN GOLDBERG

The study of parent-infant interaction in families with prematurely born infants is a relatively new endeavor. Indeed, intensive follow-ups of preterm infants were not possible until medical technology was able to ensure the survival of a large proportion of infants born prematurely. The early follow-ups (e.g., Drillien 1964) were concerned primarily with the physical and mental development of infants, and the caregiving environment, if studied at all, was assessed in global terms (e.g., socioeconomic status, parent attitudes) and was of interest for its potential effects on physical and intellectual growth. This parallels a similar orientation in the broader area of infant development, where the primary focus was on cognition. The caregiving environment was of interest only insofar as it might influence the development of cognitive skills.

Research on the Development of Prematurely Born Infants

The traditional approach to studying the sequelae of prematurity assumed a mechanistic model of development. An event occurring at time *t* was assumed to be the "cause" of something in the child's behavior at a later time $t + n$. Investigators accordingly searched for correlations between specific early events or measurements (e.g., gestational age, birth weight, Apgar scores) and later functioning (most often on IQ tests). As the evidence accumulated, it became increasingly clear that, from a practical point of view, events in the neonatal period were rather unsuccessful predictors of later development (Parmelee & Haber 1973).

In a chapter published in 1975, Sameroff and Chandler reviewed the literature and made several important points. First, they concluded that characteristics of the enduring caregiving environment seemed to be more potent predictors of developmental outcomes than were isolated early events. Second, they summarized evidence which indicated that characteristics of the infant can affect the quality of the caregiving environment. Finally, they argued for a more complex model of development, which they termed "transactional." In such a model, development can only be predicted on a short-term basis from multiple measures of infant and environmental characteristics in the immediately preceding period. Development is a series of states, each of which is multiply influenced by prior states and exerts influences on immediately subsequent states.

This more complex model suggests that in order to study the development of the preterm infant in a way which allows prediction of specific outcomes, it is necessary to make repeated assessments of many factors for both the infant and the environment. The infant-caregiver relationship is one of these factors, and more recent follow-ups of prematurely born infants have adopted a repeated assessment strategy and included interaction measures (e.g., Field et al. 1978 found that interactive measures were essential in distinguishing preterm infants continuing at risk from those who were developing normally).

In summary, there have been two reasons for studying parent-infant interaction among dyads with preterm infants. One is to develop more effective predictors of developmental outcomes for preterm infants. The second is to provide a better understanding of the development of parent-child relationships by exploring similarities and differences between dyads with differing early experiences. The next section will focus primarily on studies motivated by the latter considerations.

Parent-Infant Interaction in Preterm Dyads

The studies to be reviewed in this section are those which made comparisons between preterm and full-term dyads and/or between preterm dyads with differing early experiences. Virtually all of these studies excluded infants who were small for dates or had known congenital defects.

The very first studies in this area were concerned with the extent to which contact with the infant affected the initiation and maintenance of maternal behavior. Until the 1960s, routine care for preterm infants separated them from their parents for most, if not all, of their hospitalization. In part, this reflected a concern for minimizing infections by allowing only essential (and well-scrubbed) personnel into the intensive care unit. Concern for the possible detrimental effects of such practices on maternal behavior motivated a group of researchers at Stanford University Medical Center to take the (then) daring step of allowing parents into the premature nursery to handle their babies (Barnett et al. 1970). They were able to demonstrate the feasibility of introducing such practices without increasing infections, and in some sense this made possible all of the research to be discussed here.

A subsequent study at Stanford made comparisons between three groups: normal full-term dyads, preterm dyads receiving routine hospital care (separation group), and preterm dyads in which mothers were allowed to handle the infants while they were still in incubators (control group). Nursery procedures were varied for set time periods so that all preterm infants in the nursery during a given period received the same treatment. It was expected that the extra interactive experience in the contact group would lead to maternal behavior more similar to that of the full-term group than the separated preterm group.

This and other early studies which were initially concerned with effects of separation do suggest that separation may contribute to interactive differences between full-term and preterm dyads. However, the contact manipulation and its effects were relatively weak.

Probably because these early studies were concerned with the effects of exposure to infants on mothers, little data are given concerning infant behavior during the interactions described. While the authors suggest that separation or lack of interactive experience contributed to a lowered level of participation and self-confidence among preterm mothers, it is possible that this might also have been a response to characteristic features of the infants' behavior.

A more recent study of preterm infants seems to suggest that separation *per se* may contribute less to differences between full-term and preterm dyads than problematic infant behavior. Field (1977a) compared face-to-face interaction of mothers with 3½-month-olds in three groups: full-term infants, preterms who had experienced respiratory distress, and post-mature infants. Both the preterm and the post-mature babies had received poor scores on the interactive scales of the Brazelton Neonatal Behavior Assessment scales (Brazelton 1973), but only the preterm infants had experienced prolonged separation from parents. However, in face-to-face play, both preterm and post-mature babies were more inattentive than the full-term group. At the same time, mothers of the preterm and post-mature babies were more active than mothers in the full-term group. Thus, parents of both preterm and post-mature babies worked harder than parents of full-term infants, but were less successful in getting their infants' attention. However, all infants were more attentive when parents were given instructions which led to lowered activity rates (i.e., "try to imitate your baby's behavior"). This suggests that although infant inattention may have initially stimulated parents to increase their activity, the increased activity level led to infant inattention. Thus, both level of infant attention and parent activity contributed to the quality of the interaction.

The finding that preterm infants are behaviorally more difficult social partners is corroborated by other studies. DiVitto and Goldberg (1979) used the Brazelton scales to evaluate four groups of infants before hospital discharge: full-term infants, healthy preterm infants, sick (respiratory distress) preterm infants, and preterm infants of diabetic mothers. The first three groups showed a consistent ordering such that the full-term infants consistently obtained better scores than the healthy preterms, who scored better than the sick preterm group.

Like Field (1977a), DiVitto and Goldberg (1979) also found that scores on the Brazelton scales were related to later interactions, in this case, feeding behavior in the first four months. Infants who were alert and responsive during the neonatal assessment were more alert and looked at their parents more during feedings. Babies who had been unresponsive and difficult to rouse during the neonatal examination received more functional stimulation (e.g., nipple movement) during feedings than babies who were responsive and easy to rouse. Thus, parents of unresponsive babies were more active (i.e., worked harder) than those whose babies readily engaged in the task at hand. However, at the two newborn feedings, the full-term infants were held closer, touched, and talked to more than any of the preterm groups. Brown and Bakeman (1979) also observed feedings of full-term and preterm infants at one and three months post-discharge. As the authors describe it, mothers of preterm infants "carried more of the interactive burden" than mothers of full-term infants.

The tendency of parents to be more active with more problematic infants is supported by the observations of Beckwith and Cohen (1978). In a sample of 123 preterm infants, the relationship between obstetric and postnatal complications and caregiver–infant interaction at one month was evaluated. Those infants who had experienced more obstetric and postnatal medical complications received more frequent caregiving and more social and verbal stimulation. Unlike the others, this study did not look at detailed interactions in a standard setting but used a lengthy home observation that included a variety of potential caregiving and social interactions.

Few studies have examined interactions of preterm infants and parents beyond the early months, but one study has followed interactions in the second half of the first year. Brachfeld and Goldberg (1978) have observed the infants in the DiVitto and

Goldberg (1979) study at 8 and 12 months in a play situation both in the home and in the laboratory. Four toys were provided, and parents were asked to interact with the infant on the floor as they normally would (including not interacting if it seemed appropriate). At eight months, infants in the sick preterm group played least and fussed most of all four groups, while their parents were most active of all groups in staying close, touching their babies, and offering and demonstrating toys. In contrast, the full-term infants spent more time in play, fussed the least, smiled most, and had parents who were least active and smiled most of the four groups. The healthy preterm group was most similar to the full-term group, while infants of diabetic mothers were most similar to the sick preterm group. These group differences were no longer present at the 12-month assessments.

Summary and Implications

These studies, though few in number and different in purpose and method, do seem to provide some fairly consistent evidence of differences in parent-infant interaction as a function of neonatal medical problems. Those studies which have assessed the infant as a potential social partner in the neonatal period (DiVitto & Goldberg 1979; Field 1977a; 1977b) reported that preterm infants were less alert and responsive to social stimulation than their full-term counterparts. Observations of very early interactions of parents with full-term and preterm infants indicate that parents of preterm infants are less actively involved with their babies than parents in full-term dyads. Relative to parents of full-term infants, parents of prematures made less body contact (DiVitto & Goldberg 1979; Klaus et al. 1970; Leifer et al. 1972), spent less time face-to-face (Klaus et al. 1970), smiled at their infants less (Leifer et al. 1972), touched them less (DiVitto & Goldberg 1979; Klaus et al. 1970; Leifer et al. 1972) and talked to them less (DiVitto & Goldberg 1979).

Those studies which have observed older infants with their parents find that where there are differences between full-term and preterm dyads, parents in the preterm dyads are more active rather than less. In most cases, this is coupled with less active or less appropriate participation on the part of the infant.

Under normal conditions, both parents and infants appear to have a full repertoire of behaviors that are well adapted for social interactions (Stern 1974a). The studies reviewed here suggest that premature birth disrupts the normal development of interactive skills for both parent and infant. At the time of hospital discharge, preterm infants were less alert and responsive and made fewer demands (by crying) for adult attention than full-term infants. These characteristics which make the young preterm infant a more difficult social partner may reflect immaturity, lack of "normal" social experiences while in the hospital, or the consequences of repeated "aversive" interactions during routine intensive care procedures (e.g., tube feeding, repeated drawing of blood samples). For the parent, the early arrival of the infant can occur before the parent is psychologically (and practically) ready for parenthood. Parents are likely to have less positive delivery experiences with this disruption of their plans and must then confront feelings of failure and grief for the full-term child they did not produce (Klaus & Kennell 1976). In addition, there are anxieties about the infant's health and survival and a prolonged period with few opportunities to engage in social interaction with their baby. Thus, in the neonatal period, social interactions in preterm dyads are less active than those in full-term dyads.

As the baby grows older, and has been home longer, these initial disadvantages may become less important and more regular patterns of interaction are established. Perhaps in response to these early difficulties, perhaps because they perceive their parental task as more important and challenging than that of the average parent, perhaps because their infants remain less responsive, parents of preterm infants seem to adopt a strategy in which they invest more time and energy in interactions than is usual in full-term dyads. It is not necessarily a consistently effective strategy. Field (1977a) found that when parents were less active their babies were more attentive rather than less. Brachfeld and Goldberg (1978) found that their sick preterm infants continued to fuss in spite of parents' active efforts to distract and/or comfort them. Nevertheless, given the early limitations of preterm infants and their parents, the more active role of these parents may serve an adaptive function.

Most of these studies focus on infants under the age of four months. Data for older infants are notably scarce. Brachfeld and Goldberg (1978) found differences between preterm and full-term infants at 8 months but not at 12 months. Leiderman and Seashore (1975) reported few differences at 11–15 months. While these findings suggest that the differences may disappear by the end of the first year, additional data seem necessary before such a conclusion can be drawn with confidence.

In considering the potential implications of these research findings, it is important to bear in mind that group differences in interactive style do not necessarily mean that one is "better" and the other "worse." These studies indicate that it is usual for preterm dyads to develop different interaction patterns than full-term dyads. Patterns which might be worrisome in a full-term dyad (e.g., delayed body contact) can be part of the typical pattern in preterm groups. Thus, before instituting efforts to make preterm dyads more like full-term dyads, we should ask, given a specific situation, does a particular pattern appear to serve an adaptive function? In the author's own study, during feedings, parents of preterm infants made repeated efforts to wake their babies and to stimulate sucking when the infant was drowsy. Parents of full-term infants were more likely to allow the baby to fall asleep and terminate the feeding. One could conclude that the parents in the preterm group "failed" to respond to the baby's signal. However, given the importance of early nutritional intake for these babies, we can also conclude that the parent responded quite appropriately to the signal by rousing the baby and making more intensive efforts to stimulate further sucking.

In recent years, hospital practices have changed considerably so that there are now few hospitals which do not allow parents to visit their infants during hospitalization. The amount of support and encouragement and the amount of parent participation considered desirable varies widely from one hospital to another. Among the studies reviewed, the amount of early contact varies considerably; yet this does not seem to contribute to differences in the findings. The sample in Boston, where the most intensive visiting occurred, does not differ markedly from the others in interactive patterns. The investigators at Stanford and Case Western Reserve, who were most interested in the effects of early contact, found little effect on parent-infant interaction. Because these early studies were innovative in introducing nursery visiting, hospital staff members had little to guide them in helping parents in this role. This may account for the low visiting rate and the apparently weak effects of the contact conditions. The current evidence seems to indicate that differences between full-term and preterm dyads are found regardless of the amount of early contact experienced.

9

Perinatal Indicators and Psychophysiological Precursors of Crib Death

LEWIS P. LIPSITT

Crib death, or the sudden infant death syndrome (SIDS), takes perhaps as many as 10,000 babies a year in the United States alone. If is the single most common "cause" of death in the first year of life, excluding the especially hazardous first few days after birth. The peak incidence is between the ages of two and four months of age, and there is seasonal variation, with peaks in the winter or spring for the United States. 90 percent of crib death cases occur before six months of age, and 99 percent before one year. Almost every case of sudden infant death syndrome occurs during a sleep period, and the infants are usually found in the morning after no apparent sign of struggle. Babies who succumb to crib death simply stop breathing, at least as far as most later inquiries can determine. There is usually no evidence of any agonal experience, no sign of pain or struggle. Interestingly, and undoubtedly significantly, a mild upper respiratory infection is found in 40 to 50 percent of the cases, with the parents reporting a runny nose, raspy breathing, and so on. There is seldom any fever. The baby has been regarded in the few days immediately preceding the death as essentially normal.

The fallout from crib death in grief, despair, and loneliness among the thousands of close survivors is a further tragedy, especially in the absence of definitive answers regarding the basic mechanisms underlying SIDS. Crib death may be properly regarded as a public health menace in terms of the numbers of persons grievously affected by it.

Although there has been a shroud of mystery associated with SIDS which has tended to preclude the avid investigation of its causes, some investigators in recent years have been able to document psychophysiological conditions which are correlated with SIDS. While the mechanisms and processes underlying crib death are not by any means clear at this time, there are tempting signs on the scientific horizon to suggest that a better understanding of the phenomenon is not far off. Steinschneider (1976), for example, has been showing persistently that apnea, or the spontaneous interruption of respiration, is a significant factor in the origins of SIDS. He believes that those infants who are particularly prone to apneic conditions during sleep are those who subsequently succumb to crib death. Thoman, Miano, and Freese (1976) have also presented data suggesting that a respiratory anomaly is involved.

Recent evidence of Emery and his colleagues in England (Protestos et al. 1973), of Naeye, Ladis, and Drage (1976), and of Anderson and Rosenblith (1971) support the respiration aberration hypothesis. Those infants who subsequently die of sudden infant death syndrome, while ostensibly normal according to most visible criteria of infant well-being, have endured histories of obstetrical/perinatal/neonatal stresses which could dispose them to "unexplained death" two or three months hence, and which do implicate respiratory problems.

We have data from a retrospective study of crib deaths in Providence, Rhode Island, which further support the proposition that respiratory abnormalities were present at birth, months before the infants died. The data to be presented here (Lipsitt, Sturner, & Burke 1979), like those of Naeye, Ladis, and Drage (1976), contribute to a picture of crib death as a subtle debility which apparently sets the stage for the later development of a specific breathing deficit. The thesis I will propose is that perinatal hazards and congenital debilities of the fetus and newborn may place the infant in special jeopardy, in that any early behavioral deficits will be compounded by the failure of experience to prepare the infant for later threats to its survival. Infants who as newborns are incapable of responding defensively to stimulus hazards will be especially vulnerable at later ages, e.g., at two to four months of age, by which time the infant must learn certain defensive postures and respiratory responses that will reduce the threats to survival from smothering or suffocation. The proposition presented here is that crib death might be a learning disability secondary to a congenital incapacity to properly divert threats to respiratory occlusion. First, the constitutional aspects of crib death:

In one recent study of the developmental histories of crib death (Naeye, Ladis, & Drage 1976), 125 SIDS victims were compared with matched controls. The data for this study were from the Collaborative Perinatal Project of the National Institute of Neurological and Communicative Disorders and Stroke in which eleven cities throughout the nation were represented. The targets of study were all born between 1959 and 1966. The investigators compared the 125 SIDS cases with over 50,000 infants of the Collaborative Study who were born alive and survived the early months of life. This "unmatched control group" was supplemented by another "matched control group" of 375 infants, matched with the victims for place of birth, date of delivery, gestational age, sex, race, and socioeconomic status. All of the matched controls were "survivors." Infants with major congenital anomalies were excluded both in the SIDS and the matched control categories.

The study found multiple signs of possible neonatal brain dysfunction in future SIDS victims. Abnormalities were documented in respiration, feeding, temperature regulation, and specific neurologic tests. Apgar scores were significantly lower in the future victims. There was a greater incidence of maternal influenza and cigarette smoking in the histories of infants who succumbed, a finding also of Bergman and Wiesner (1976). SIDS victims, moreover, had a greater proportion of young mothers of low socioeconomic and educational level, who lived in crowded housing, and who had minimal prenatal care. In the Naeye et al. study, a greater proportion of the SIDS victims were underweight at birth for gestational age. There was little or no suggestion in the histories of any hereditary influence predisposing to crib death. It was noted by Naeye et al. that many of the crib death victims who grew normally prenatally were growth-retarded following birth, probably not as a result of undernutrition.

The Naeye et al. study was a very large investigation based upon the computerized medical records of thousands of births occurring across the country. One may question whether such differences between SIDS and control cases would appear in smaller, "local" groups of potential SIDS victims and under conditions in which the SIDS victims are matched one-for-one with the next birth of the same sex and race occurring in the same hospital. Such a study was undertaken in Providence. The epidemiological or actuarial statistics relating paranatal characteristics to later crib death are borne out by a study (Lipsitt, Sturner, & Burke 1979) of the 15 crib death cases in the Providence sample of the National Collaborative Perinatal Project. Studying the 15 Providence cases (of 4,000 births) diagnosed by Naeye as true crib deaths, the Providence group confirmed that there were pathological precursors which could provide the basis for a predictive scale of developmental jeopardy in relation to SIDS, even during the newborn period. Neonatal psychophysiological factors, it was concluded, might well be involved in the final pathway to the condition that ultimately causes the death of the infant, usually between two and four months of age. By psychophysiological factors is meant not only simply autonomic nervous system deficiency, although that would be part of the story, but the effects which early experiences may have on the very young child and which experiences may affect the child's later ability to cope with stressful stimulation.

We began with the records of those 15 true SIDS cases identified by Naeye, and then selected a control group of cases which was comprised of the very next birth, of the same sex, into the project. The child was born in the same hospital, usually on the same day as the target or deceased case. We compared this control group with the SIDS group and immediately found that a second control group was required, for while there were seven infants in the deceased group that "were non-Caucasian, there were *two* in the "matched" control group. A third cohort was therefore identified, this consisting of the subsequent births into the study of both the same sex and race. The apparent relevance of race as a determinative variable in crib death, replicating the high incidence of SIDS in black children found in the much larger Naeye study, constitutes a noteworthy finding in itself.

It turned out that the deceased group varied from the controls in several ways, all of them in a direction connoting perinatal distress or biological hazard. The Apgar-score data taken from the delivery room records of the 15 SIDS cases in comparison with those of each of the control groups indicated that the SIDS group's scores were lower at each of the three times tested than the scores of either of the controls (1, 2, and 5 minutes postpartum), and that the SIDS group at 5 minutes old barely reached the level of the controls as tested at one minute of age. The differences in Apgar scores between the SIDS group and both controls were reliable at one minute, and at five minutes a reliable difference still existed between the SIDS group and Control-I.

There occurred interesting and suggestive differences between the SIDS group and the two control groups in maternal anemia during pregnancy (twice as frequent in SIDS than in the survivors), in neonatal respiratory abnormalities noted, in the need for intensive care, and in diagnosed atelectasis. The eventual SIDS victims also had lowered birth weights and body lengths, were hospitalized significantly longer than the controls, and had serum bilirubin levels reliably higher on average than those of their controls.

It seems clear that the infants who ultimately succumbed at 2, 3, 4, or 5 months of age were already showing, in general and on average, that they were beginning life with some fragility. We need to know more about that, and about the developmental processes that transform seemingly minor insufficiencies into a morbid crisis a few months later. I use the term "minor insufficiencies" advisedly, for the literature on crib death in professional journals and in public documents tends to emphasize the prior *normality* of SIDS victims. It appears that while SIDS victims are essentially normal infants, as a group they do seem to be a "risk population" that can be identified on the basis of their biographies. Better record-keeping and more intensive documentation of the perinatal histories of infants reveals a higher incidence of developmental aberration in such infants than has often been realized.

The term crib death and SIDS are in fact diagnoses of essential ignorance, which is to say that the labels are applied when no *discernible* sign of pathology in the deceased infant is present. The terms are temporizing diagnoses. They would be more useful if it were generally appreciated that the diagnosis really means that the cause of the death is not *yet* known. Research into the causes of crib death proceeds slowly.

Because of the heavy investment in pathological causation in relation to SIDS, psychophysiological theories and suppositions have not yet been sufficiently explored. Infants whose developmental histories have placed them in jeopardy, so that they require special resuscitative efforts, have lowered Apgar scores, and must remain in the hospital longer, must be assumed to have suffered some anoxic insult that is likely to subdue their activity. When infants move less, are less visually alert, feel less, suck weakly, and generally engage their environment less, they subject themselves to fewer opportunities for learning than "normal" infants do. In short, it is quite possible that the constellation of pathological signs found in the histories of SIDS cases is exactly such as to place them in special jeopardy from a learning deficiency.

The period immediately following birth is one of rapid myelinization and dendritic proliferation, and this period may be an especially important one for critical learning events. Many of the unconditioned responses with which infants come into the world, such as the rooting reflex, the Babinski and Babkin responses, the grasping reflex, and others, undergo marked changes between birth and about two months of age. It is not impossible that humans are biologically equipped to engage in certain vital responses at birth which will diminish with the passage of time, to be supplanted by learned response systems. These learned responses become increasingly important while their ontogenetic forebears diminish in frequency and vigor.

It is well known that many innate response systems which are strikingly apparent at birth and soon after (e.g., the grasping reflex, the Babkin response, primitive reaching responses, and obligatory visual attention) do diminish in their frequency and intensity with the passage of time up to around two or three months of age (Paine 1976). The firm grasp reflex, for instance, becomes a slow exploratory mode of behavior in response to the sudden pressure of an object on the palm of the hand. At least some of these response propensities are later displaced by "voluntary" learned responses mediated by higher cortical centers, perhaps in contrast to the brain-stem control that existed before experience could superimpose itself upon the lower brain function. Much brain tissue maturation occurs shortly after birth, particularly in the first two months of human life (Dobbing 1975; Purpura 1975), and it may well be that this period of development is in some respects critical for the experiential accretion of certain learned responses. Could it not be that if some behavioral patterns are inadequately learned by a certain age, coinciding with the time by which the unlearned protective reflexes have diminished to an ineffective level, the organism will not have been prepared adequately for survival?

The "natural" defensive response of the normal neonate to respiratory occlusion, or even to the *threat* of occlusion as imposed by the presence of a covering over a part of the baby's face (as in Brazelton's scale) is for a series of defensive actions to be taken. These have been described by Lipsitt (1976), in part after a description of the pediatrician Gunther (1955, 1961) who observed such struggling of newborns while suckling at the breast. The response pattern is rather like an enraged response which escalates as the stimulus is prolonged. At birth and in the intact organism, the behavior pattern is essentially fail-safe, culminating in crying and ultimately freeing the respiratory passages (Graham 1976).

If the newborn does not have a strong defensive response to threats to respiration, or to head restraint, it is possible that the appropriate voluntary operant behaviors which must ultimately supplant this congenital response by around two months of age will not be learned.

This supposition seems to have validity as a hypothesis, both in terms of the circumstances usually surrounding crib death and in consideration of data already available. There is good evidence, some just presented, that crib death cases have, as a group, begun life with some organismic deficits associated with perinatal stresses. Infants who succumb in the first year of life without any obvious fatal disease are demonstrably, as a group, mildly deficient in their responses to respiratory occlusion at birth or are in some other respect behaviorally lethargic (Anderson & Rosenblith 1971). Moreover, the data of Steinschneider (1976), of Thoman, Miano, and Freese (1976), and others, point to respiratory anomalies in many histories of crib death and near-miss cases.

Crib death occurs mostly at night while others are sleeping. Such deaths are more frequent in the winter and spring months. Lower socioeconomic families are at greatest risk generally, and a cold or "sniffles" had usually been observed in the deceased infant in the few days prior to the death. Respiratory occlusion, failure of appropriate defensive behavior, and inadequate compensatory mouth-breathing when the nostrils are clogged could conceivably lead to anoxia and a comatose state, and ultimately to the infant's death, particularly when all of these conditions converge as in sleeping infants with a cold and a history of insufficient response to threatening stimulation. Such a pathway to death might involve no agonal responses whatever, as the eventual death might well have occurred in a comatose child.

It is quite possible that infants who have not learned to engage in the responses necessary for clearing the respiratory passages or clearing the way *to* those passages when threatened with occlusion will be those in particular jeopardy at the critical ages of two to four months.

While I am suggesting, then, that crib death may be a developmental disability involving a learning deficit, I hope that I will not be misunderstood to be saying that the cause of crib death *is* a learning disorder. My position is that, in the absence of substantial data in support of other hypotheses, and in view of the present evidence that these infants begin life under hazardous conditions and have response aberrations, there is a reasonable possibility of learning dysfunction. Such an anomaly could place disposed infants in special jeopardy between two and four months of age, when there is a marked developmental transition from involuntary reflexive functioning in many sensory motor modalities to responding on a voluntary, deliberative, and learned basis mediated by increasing cortical control.

I wish to be clearly understood in regard to the nature of the posited learning aberration. No human response system of which I am aware could be classified as either solely constitutional or totally experiential. To the extent that a learning anomaly is in part responsible for the demise of crib-death infants, I would still want to insist upon the congenital or constitutional deficit as well. No learning process can take place without the prior presence of a constitutional system that supports, and in its origin provides the permission for, the learned response to occur. Thus it is my position that there must have been a congenital response deficit present at the outset, which provided the setting condition for the deficient respiratory occlusion response to manifest itself. To the extent that weak defensive reflexes are found at birth in these susceptible infants, the development of learned responses necessary for the infant to retrieve its respiratory passages for breathing when threatened with occlusion is compromised.

PART III

Cognitive-Perceptual Development

Ever since the Russians beat the United States into space with the launching of Sputnik in the 1950s, there has been what can only be described as an explosion of interest in cognitive development in American developmental psychology. Policy makers realized that if America was to successfully compete with the Soviet Union, talents would have to be nurtured early and that, if this were to be accomplished, a basic understanding of the development of intellectual ability would be required. Thus was born one powerful force that led to the emphasis on cognitive development in American psychology.

A second force lay in the promises of the 1960s and the push for a Great Society that would eliminate poverty in American culture. For out of this movement came the early Head Start programs that strove to enhance the cognitive and physical functioning of children from high risk environments in hopes of eliminating the school failure that children from such contexts were known to display and which was considered to contribute to the intergenerational transmission of poverty. Again, a basic understanding of intellectual growth was recognized to be a prerequisite if these early efforts to enhance individual development, and therby enhance society, were to succeed.

That such forces in American society proved successful in stimulating advances in our understanding of early cognitive functioning owes as much to the long unnoticed work of Piaget as to the historical context itself. For without Piaget's seminal theory of cognitive development, much of which had been detailed decades earlier, it is not at all certain that the progress which has been made over the past 15 to 20 years would have been possible. Piaget provided a focal point, that is, a perspective or approach that could be agreed with or disagreed with but which, in any event, could be examined empirically. With such a foundation, developmentalists set out to test the validity of Piaget's claims, and the cognitive revolution began.

Some of the fruits of that revolution are illustrated in the essays included in this section. In the first, Leslie Cohen makes an overview of "Our Developing Knowledge of Infant Perception and Cognition" and demonstrates how and why our ideas regarding the infant have changed since the time when William James described the baby's world as a "booming, buzzing confusion." Indeed, today we speak of the "competent infant" who not only perceives stimuli from the time of birth onward, but who also can discriminate between colors, shapes, and forms, and display preferences from among them.

As Cohen also points out, this developing knowledge regarding the information that the infant perceives or "picks up" has important implications for our understanding of higher order cognitive processes and the early diagnoses of handicapping conditions. For example, the fact that young infants habituate (i.e., stop responding) to repeatedly presented events (e.g., picture of a ball), but will reinitiate responding when a new stimuli is offered (e.g., picture of a cube), demonstrates that the child at so early an age possesses the capacity for memory. A knowledge of early individual differences in these and other skills may someday allow us to identify early on children who may have subsequent perceptual or learning disabilities. To the extent that this possibility proves true, the implications for early intervention are profound. For as Cohen points out, efforts to remediate problems before they create serious handicaps can then become possible.

This brief discussion of the diagnostic potential of early assessments of perceptual abilities underscores one of the enduring themes that motivate infancy researchers—the relationship of early functioning and later development. In the second article in this section, McCall and his colleagues take up this issue as part of their effort to examine changes in the nature of infant sensorimotor development across the first two years of life. Drawing upon a large longitudinal data set, these investigators document transformation in early mental functioning and measure the predictive power of early tests. With respect to this latter issue, they accurately note that, with the exception of severely impaired performance during the infancy years, performance on standardized developmental tests during the first stage of life are not very powerful predictors of later cognitive skill.

The reason for this finding, McCall et al. argue, is that early infant intelligence undergoes epigenetic transformation (i.e., qualitative changes) so that what underlies performance at one age does not necessarily do so at a later period. This does not mean, however, that no relationships exist across developmental periods. For, in fact, the study which these investigators report reveals some stability in individual differences. When total scores derived from standardized tests are statistically decomposed into subsets, meaningful relations emerge between early and later performance, beginning as early as 6 months of age.

Probably more intriguing than this finding, however, is the qualitative change in sensorimotor functioning that McCall and his colleagues uncover across infant test performance at 6, 12, 18, and 24 months when total scores are decomposed. At 6 months, early cognitive skill is found to involve primarily minipulative exploration of objects that produce perceptual contingencies (e.g., bang spoon on table to make sound), a process that strongly resembles Piaget's notion of secondary circular reaction. At 12 months, elementary verbal behavior, especially in a social context, and the imitation of rudimentary social skills (e.g., waving bye-bye) are identified. Cognitive skill becomes increasingly verbal in character by the end of the first half of the second year, and this trend continues, McCall et al. note, through 24 months, with infants showing ever-increasing ability to both generate and understand spoken language.

The transformational character of early cognitive or sensorimotor skill which Piaget's theory prescribes, and which McCall et al. uncovered in infant test data, is also evident in Belsky and Most's study of infant free play behavior. Indeed, their article strongly suggests, as Piaget, again, noted long ago, that infant exploration/play can serve as a "window" on cognitive development. What is most interesting about these data is the light they shed upon the ontogeny of early manipulative activity. In the last quarter of the first year, different objects tend to be treated very much alike, being mouthed, turned over, or banged, and only gradually does the infant come to exploit the unique properties of a toy. Once such exploration succeeds in teaching the child about the parts of an object, he becomes able to include the toy as a prop in pretend play. Such pretense activity itself undergoes development so that the child eventually becomes able to substitute props in his play, and to put pretense acts together to create little stories (e.g., drink from minature cup and wipe mouth with piece of green felt, used as a napkin).

It has been suggested that the development of such play skill is programmed by the same underlying cognitive structure that is responsible for language development, since both domains of behavior require skill in using symbols. But it is important to note, as Spieker does in the last article in this section, that the precursors of language are evident long before children begin to engage in pretense play. In fact, Spieker shows in her overview of the development of language during infancy that infants may learn rules about communication that are essential to language use long before they sound their first words. The nature of the child's early interactions with its caregiver provides a context for learning language and may even determine, as Spieker also shows, what words the child first uses and the kinds of sentences he eventually makes. The main point of Spieker's presentation is that language development begins long before the child speaks and remains one of the most complicated, most studied, yet least understood psychological phenomenon that developmental psychologists have set their minds to.

10

Our Developing Knowledge of Infant Perception and Cognition

LESLIE B. COHEN

Over the past two decades, the study of infant development has progressed more rapidly than many other types of research. Although there has been a broad-based and dramatic expansion in research on social, language, cognitive, and perceptual development during this period, I would propose that one of the leading areas, if not the leading area, in this advancement has been infant perception. More has been learned about infant perception in the past fifteen or twenty years than in all previous years. Many generations have been interested in infant perceptual abilities. As early as 1877, Darwin thrust a candle before his infant son's eyes to test his vision and found him able to fixate. Darwin also noticed that sneezing or producing other unexpected noises elicited a startle response. Other isolated studies of infant perception (e.g., Chase 1937; Cruickshank 1941; Ling 1941; Valentine 1913–1914) appeared throughout the early twentieth century. It was not until Fantz's pioneering work in the late 1950s and early 1960s, however, that research in the area accelerated dramatically. Fantz's early contribution stemmed as much or more from the method he used as from the stimuli he presented or the results he obtained. His work demonstrated that one can simply and reliably measure infant visual fixations. All one must do is present some visual target, look through a peephole at the infant's eye, and record the amount of time the target is reflected on the infant's cornea (Fantz 1961). In other words, Fantz devised a simple technique for measuring infant visual perception.

The study of infant perception is intriguing in that infants cannot be asked to express exactly what they are seeing, hearing, or feeling. Yet, as Darwin reported so long ago, young infants do react to external stimulation. They must therefore be perceiving something. The question is: Just what are they perceiving? Our natural curiosity about infants, coupled with a viable technique for investigating infant perception, provided the impetus needed for the inauguration of research in this area.

Shortly after the introduction of Fantz's technique, numerous investigators, with a limited amount of inexpensive equipment and little or no prior experience with infants, began to use his procedure to study infant visual perception and cognition. Many used what has become known as the "infant preference" technique (Berlyne 1958; Fantz 1958). On each trial, two visual stimuli were presented simultaneously and infants' responses to the stimuli were compared. Actually, all that was usually recorded was the total fixation time to each stimulus. Although some considered this procedure too crude and devised more sophisticated electronic systems for tracking individual eye movements in newborns (Salapatek 1968), others made ingenious use of this simple procedure ("show them some pictures and see which one they like the most") to examine everything from visual acuity to intermodal coordination. In some of Fantz's earlier work, for example, he showed that infants prefer to look longer at a patterned surface than at a plain one (Fantz 1963). This simple fact has been used in numerous investigations of the development of infant visual acuity (Fantz, Ordy, & Udelf 1962; Salapatek, Bechtold, & Buchnell 1976). One can put vertical black and white stripes on one side and a plain grey stimulus on the other. By decreasing the contrast of the lines or by increasing their spatial frequency, one can determine at what point the infants' preference (and presumably their ability to discriminate between patterned and unpatterned stimuli) disappears. Although actual estimates of infant visual acuity vary somewhat from study to study, we do know that the newborn's acuity is quite poor but that it increases dramatically during the first few months of life (Cohen, DeLoache, & Strauss 1979). This knowledge and simple procedure are now beginning to be used on an applied basis in some hospitals to diagnose infants with suspected visual defects (Dobson et al. 1978).

In some ways, studies of visual acuity may be considered the limiting case of studies of visual preference. They test whether the infants see something or nothing. Of equal interest are those experiments that present two different perceivable stimuli and test whether or not infants can discriminate between them. Numerous experiments of this sort have shown infant preferences for curved versus straight lines (Fantz & Nevis 1967; Ruff & Birch 1974), chromatic versus achromatic stimuli (Fantz 1963; Oster 1975), three-dimensional objects versus two-dimensional representations (Fantz, Fagan, & Miranda 1975), complex patterns versus simple ones (Brennan, Ames, & Moore 1966; Fantz 1965), and schematic faces versus nonfaces (Fantz 1963; Goren 1975). One of the most ingenious recent uses of the technique was devised by Spelke (1978) in the study of intermodal perception. Four-month-old infants were simultaneously shown two films: one of a bouncing toy kangaroo and one of a bouncing donkey. The filmed objects each moved at a different rate. From a central speaker, the infants heard the sound appropriate to one of the films. Spelke found that the infants looked significantly longer at the film associated with the sound, thus demonstrating the ability to coordinate auditory and visual information. In a refinement of this procedure in our laboratory, Maynard (1979) showed the identical jumping-kangaroo film on both sides. The only difference between the films was that they were temporally out of phase. Once again, a central speaker produced a sound appropriate to one of the films. Four-month-old males looked significantly longer at the appropriate film, indicating intermodal coordination based solely on the synchrony between auditory and visual information.

As valuable as the visual preference paradigm has proven to be, it does have one inherent drawback. Its effectiveness depends on the infant having greater inborn or automatic preferences for some stimuli. When such a preference occurs, one can use it to infer the infant's ability to discriminate between stimuli, but there are innumerable instances when the infant may be able to discriminate between patterns or objects but does not have any initial preference for one over the other. Once again, we turn to Fantz for the solution of this problem. In addition to infants having a visual preference for certain characteristics of physical stimuli, Fantz reported that infants also have a preference for a novel versus a familiar stimulus (Fantz 1964). Fantz obtained evidence for novelty preference in the following cleverly designed experiment: On one side of a display screen he presented the same visual pattern on every trial, and on the other side of the screen the pattern changed from trial to trial. Over the course of the experiment, the infants gradually looked longer and longer at the side with the novel pattern.

Variations of this novelty preference paradigm have proven to be even more effective tools for assessing infant perceptual discrimination than was the earlier visual preference procedure. The novelty paradigm provides the opportunity to test infants on visual discriminations even when there appears to be no a priori preference for one stimulus. Today, the most commonly used version of the paradigm involves repeatedly presenting a single stimulus until the infant's attention habituates and then testing with the same stimulus versus one or more novel stimuli to determine when recovery of attention occurs. Thus the infant is still responding in terms of a visual preference, but it is an experimentally induced preference for novelty rather than a stimulus preference that the infant brings to the experimental situation.

Within the last 10 years, the habituation or novelty preference paradigm has been employed in countless experiments. From these studies, we know infants can perceive colors, forms, patterns, faces, and even complex events such as subject-object relations (Cohen & Strauss 1979). The more the paradigm has been used, the more sophisticated the experimental questions have become. There is now evidence that within the first six months of life infants perceive colors categorically (Bornstein 1976) and perceive simple forms or angles in terms of the relations among their sides (Schwartz 1975). Furthermore, infants can perceive simple patterns as gestalts (Vurpillot, Ruel, & Castrec 1977) and perceive more complex patterns in terms of their components, until about 5 months of age, when they perceive them as compounds (Cohen & Gelber 1975).

Summarizing what we now know, the extensive literature on infant visual perception is beginning to yield a consistent picture of how the infant processes visual information during the first few months of life. During the first month or two, infants are capable of processing high-contrast, low-spatial-frequency information. The units of perception are lines, angles, and adjacent high-contrast areas. From 2 until 4 or 5 months of age, simple dimensions such as colors and forms can be processed as units. These units are defined relationally rather than as simple transformations of energy impinging on the retina. Colors are seen categorically; that is, wide ranges of reds, yellows, greens, and blues are perceived as equivalent, whereas there are sharper boundaries between these color categories. Simple forms are perceived as holistic units, that is, in terms of the relation among their parts. It is not until approximately 5 months of age, however, that more complex patterns such as faces or colored forms are perceived as higher order gestalts. This view represents quite a change from the one held a mere two decades ago, when investigators were trying to determine whether the young infant could see at all.

There is no doubt that the habituation or novelty preference paradigm has served us well in our quest for information about how the young infant perceives his or her visual world. But the paradigm has also been valuable in another respect, perhaps more valuable to psychology as a whole than many would have anticipated. In an effort to explain not only what an infant can perceive or discriminate but why the infant habituates or has a novelty preference in the first place, many infant researchers are beginning to ask questions that transcend perception and are more relevant to the early development of memory and cognition. This transition marks the first time that that hardy soul, the infant researcher, has entered the mainstream of developmental psychology and has begun to address the same issues his or her counterparts (working with children or adults) have been investigating. Exploring issues such as recall versus recognition, short-term versus long-term memory, top-down versus bottom-up processing, and the nature of the prototype in concept acquisition has become just as important to the infant researcher as it has long been to colleagues working with older subjects.

The shift to cognition really began when infant researchers began to examine seriously the fact that infant habituation implies infant memory. An infant habituates to a stimulus because the stimulus is becoming more familiar. But in order for it to be familiar, it must, in some sense, be remembered. Thus, those experiments which showed that infants preferred a novel color or form to a familiar one also showed that infants remembered the familiar color or form. One could easily do experiments to investigate how long an infant could remember, whether that memory was subject to interference, or whether the same type of information was retained in long-term as in short-term memory.

In order to study long-term memory, all one had to do was to insert a delay between the end of habituation and a subsequent test with novel and familiar stimuli. In one experiment, for example, 5-month-old infants familiarized to a face for two minutes still retained some information about that face after a two-week delay (Fagan 1973). In order to investigate interference effects, all one had to do was to insert some irrelevant material before the test, during the delay interval. Several studies have now shown that infant memory is relatively insensitive to a whole host of interfering stimuli (Cohen, DeLoache, & Pearl 1977; Fagan 1977; McCall, Kennedy, & Dodds 1977).

Although these experiments demonstrated that infant memory is robust and that information can be retained for long periods of time, research is just beginning to examine whether information retained in long-term memory is the same as or different from information retained in short-term memory. In one experiment recently completed in our laboratory (Strauss & Cohen 1978), 5-month-old infants were familiarized with a three-dimensional Styrofoam figure. They were then tested immediately, after a 10-minute delay, and after a 24-hour delay, with the same form and one with a different shape, color, size, or orientation. Although the infants exhibited recognition of all four dimensions when tested immediately, they retained only the color and form after 10 minutes and only the form after 24 hours. If one assumes that these dimensions can be arranged hierarchically according to depth of processing or salience of the dimension for knowledge about objects, with form being more salient than color, then this study provides the first evidence that infants retain longest those characteristics that are most salient or important.

One of the more exciting new developments in infant perception is adaptation of the habituation paradigm to investigate concept acquisition in the infant. According to the standard habituation procedure, the infant is repeatedly shown the same stimulus. In a concept study, the infant is shown a variety of different stimuli, all of which belong to the same concept or category, and is then tested with a new member of the category and a nonmember. If the infant has remembered the concept as opposed to the individual stimuli, his or her habituation should generalize more to the new member of category than to the nonmember. These experiments are equivalent to ones with older children in which the subjects are shown several examples from a category and are then asked to select the test items that are members of the same category. Several experiments with infants have now been reported that have used this habituation procedure. Most have used faces as stimuli (Cohen & Strauss 1979; Cornell 1974; Fagan 1974), although there is also evidence of categorization of stuffed animals (Cohen & Caputo 1978), photographs of real animals (Cohen & Caputo 1978), and shapes regardless of orientation (McGurk 1972).

From an applied perspective, our expanding knowledge about developmental changes in perception, information processing, and cognition in normal infants is an essential first step toward diagnosis and remediation of specific perceptual or cognitive deficits in high-risk or retarded infants. It is popular these days to assume that infants who have had some perinatal trauma or inadequate environment will be developmentally retarded. Intervention programs for infants are sprouting up all over the country to deal with that assumed retardation. Many of these programs are undoubtedly doing some good, yet because of our current lack of knowledge, most programs are forced to work largely in the dark. Before we can effectively remedy some perceptual or cognitive problem, we must be able to diagnose the specifics of the problem. And before we can make that diagnosis we must learn how the normal infant develops and changes. We already know enough about a few areas, such as the development of visual acuity or color vision, to make early diagnosis possible. Assuming that the current rate of research on infant perception will continue in the next few years, we are likely to achieve that same goal in the more elusive areas of early perceptual organization and cognition. A short time ago, we had to admit that the study of infant development was itself in its own infancy. Today, we can say with some pride that the study of infant development is coming of age.

11

Transitions in Infant Sensorimotor Development and the Prediction of Childhood IQ

ROBERT B. McCALL, PAMELA SAVOY HOGARTY,
AND NANCY HURLBURT

Over the last 50 years, there have been numerous attempts to relate developmental test scores, obtained during infancy, to standardized intelligence tests, given later in adolescence and adulthood. Reviews of this literature (Bayley 1970; Rutter 1970; Stott & Ball 1965; Thomas 1970) tend to concur with Bayley's summarization:

> The findings of these early studies of mental growth of infants have been repeated sufficiently often so that it is now well-established that test scores earned in the first year or two have relatively little predictive validity (in contrast to tests at school age or later), although they may have high validity as measures of the children's cognitive ability at the time [p. 1174]

The purpose of this article is twofold. First, the empirical literature concerning the prediction of childhood and adult IQ scores from infancy is reviewed, with a special focus on the possibility of psychometric factors clouding long-term prediction. Second, since most of that research was inspired by and executed under the assumption of an immutable, pervasive, general intellectual trait, the other goal of this article is to consider an alternative point of view.

Early Research

Prediction from Infancy

Normal children. It is something of an overstatement to say that there is "no prediction" from the infancy period to childhood IQ. There are correlations that attain statistical significance between certain ages for some tests, but the size of the relationships is not particularly impressive and certainly not adequate for clinical application (e.g., see table 11.1). Table 11.1 displays the median level of prediction from several ages during the first 30 months of life to childhood IQ measured between 3 and 18 years.

There are two obvious trends in the table. The first is that when predicting to any age in childhood, the later the test is given during the infancy period, the higher the relationship. Second, correlations to IQ at 3 to 4 years are higher than with IQ scores assessed thereafter.

Nonnormal samples. One purpose of developing infant tests was to detect children who might have severe pathologies. Sev-

Table 11.1 Median Correlations Between Infant Tests and Childhood IQ for Normal Children

Childhood age (yrs)	Age in Infancy Months			
	1–6	7–12	13–18	19–30
8–18	.01	.20	.21	.49
	(12/4)	(8/2)	(6/2)	(9/2)
5–7	.01	.06	.30	.41
	(7/5)	(5/4)	(5/4)	(16/4)
3–4	.23	.33	.47	.54
	(7/4)	(5/3)	(6/4)	(16/3)

NOTE: The number of correlations entering into the median and the number of different studies included are found in parentheses.

eral studies have correlated total score on infant tests with later IQ for samples involving subjects having extremely low infant test scores or subjects having known or suspected abnormalities. They indicate that prediction between infancy and childhood IQ for those infants scoring below 80 is higher than for subjects scoring above 80. Briefly, infant tests may have contemporary as well as predictive utility in identifying pathological and "suspect" conditions in infancy, and a very low score on an infant test, even though a pediatrician does not classify the child as abnormal (and vice versa), may have diagnostic value.

Some Redirection

Basic Concept of Development

The search for correlational stability across vastly different ages implies a faith in a developmentally constant, general conception of intelligence that presumably governs an enormous variety of mental activities. Under that assumption, the nature of the behavioral manifestations of "g" would change from age to age, but g itself is presumed constant, and thus mental precocity at one age should predict mental precocity at another. Confronted with the evidence reviewed above, this g model of mental development must be questioned. The following discussion emphasizes one empirical approach to developmental transitions in performance during infancy and childhood that makes somewhat less restrictive conceptual assumptions concerning mental traits and their development than many previous orientations.

It is quite likely that the several skills that characterize a given stage in infancy will vary considerably in the extent to which they share common determinants. Thus, at any specific age there might be some skills that are highly related and others that are independent. This same proposition may apply when skills are viewed *developmentally*.

The belief in an unchanging, pervasive general mental ability assumed that there was some constant determinant that governed the performance of a vast number of skills both within and across ages, and thus one should expect high within-age correlations among diverse behaviors and a single, unified, and continuous trend of relationships across age. The fact that many different abilities of childhood did show positive intercorrelations presumably testified to a single underlying dimension which then became reified under the rubric of intelligence (or g). Soon, intelligence was used to explain the very behavior that mothered its theoretical existence. The evidence for a single major mental ability either within an age—(e.g., the independent "dimensions" of Guilford (1967) or the "creativity" of Wallach and Kogan (1965)—or across age is not very convincing. However, neither do these data argue for the conceptually opposite conclusion. It seems unlikely that there are no common processes underlying some mental activities, no hierarchical organization of skills, no generality from one task to another, and no predictability from one age to another for some processes.

Consequently, one model of mental performance with heuristic value might fall somewhere between these two extremes (e.g., see Bayley 1970). First, one would suppose that within any given age (or developmental level), one could discern subsets of skills that would be highly related within a set, but the subsets would be independent from one another. Some of these skill sets might possess relationships with similar or qualitatively different skill sets at a future age; others might lead to a "dead end" in terms of their developmental significance. The matrix of developmental transitions and interactions might be quite complex.

The remainder of this essay is devoted to describing empirically such possible transitions during infancy and childhood with the purpose of illustrating this conceptual approach and generating hypotheses about the fabric of early development.

Developmental Transitions in the Fels Data

The responses of infants to individual items on Gesell tests at 6, 12, 18, and 24 months of age were subjected to principal component analyses separately at each age. The resulting components presumably represented independent skill areas within each age. Next, the component scores were correlated across age (and with childhood IQ scores) and the network of developmental transitions examined.

Subjects and analyses. The subjects were all children from the Fels population who had at least one Gesell test at either 6, 12, 18, or 24 months, and who had at least one of the following assessments in childhood: a Binet at 3½, 6, or 10 years; the WISC at 7 or 11 years; or the Wechsler-Bellevue at 13 years. Logically dependent items on the infant tests (e.g., "sits with slight support," "sits alone") were combined into a single item within each of the four Gesell segments, leaving 32, 33, 34, and 28 items on each of the four Gesell tests, respectively. The subjects' responses to these were subjected to principal components analyses separately at each age (6, 12, 18, 24 months) on the combined-sex sample (N = 158, 148, 145, 144, respectively). Separate component analyses were performed for the two sexes, but no major sex differences were found. However, while the component structure within each age did not appear different for the sexes, the correlations between component scores across age did contain sex differences (see following results).

Results. The component scores at each age were correlated. The correlation matrix is depicted graphically for boys (figure 11.1) and girls (figure 11.2). In these figures, the boxes represent components, and the number within the box indicates whether it was the first, second, etc., component extracted at that age. Shaded boxes denote that at least one correlation between this component and a childhood IQ assessment (any Binet total score, or Wechsler verbal, performance, or total score for the tests indicated above) was significant ($p < .05$, two-tailed). The numbers placed above the lines connecting boxes indicate the correlation between these two component scores, with the asterisks indicating the significance of the correlation and the triangles denoting the significance of the difference between the sexes on this correlation (asterisk or triangle signifies $p < .05$, two tailed). Boxes below the double line are components that predicted later IQ but were not involved in any significant pattern of continuity through the infancy period.

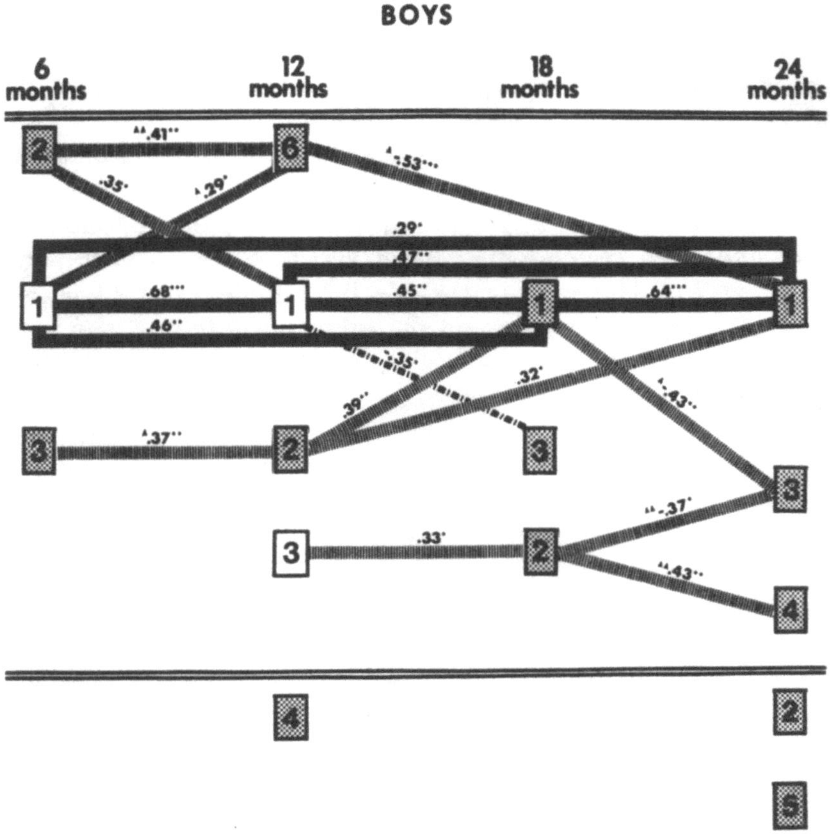

Figure 11.1 Correlation Matrix Depicted Graphically for Boys.

Figures 11.1 and 11.2 may be viewed as representing one estimate of the network of behavioral transitions that characterize infancy for boys and girls. Several general characteristics may be observed in these figures. First, each sex has a single *main developmental trend* consisting of the items loading on the first principal component at each age (connected by solid lines). The main trend was the only developmental pattern in which adjacent-age *and* nonadjacent-age correlations were both significant. While this major trend consisting of the first principal components has the appearance of a g factor, none of the components accounted for more than 19 percent of the total test variance.

Second, at 6 months, the items in the main trend do not predict childhood IQ, though some smaller components do correlate with childhood IQ. This observation has several implications. Initially it suggests that precocity in certain skills characteristic of early infancy may not relate to later childhood IQ, even though such skills may be vital precursors of those childhood traits. Further, since the main trend was composed of the first principal component at each age and since that component is presumably the best single concentrated reflection of the test as a whole, a great deal more information and predictive power may lie within subsets of items than is possessed by the total score. Moreover,

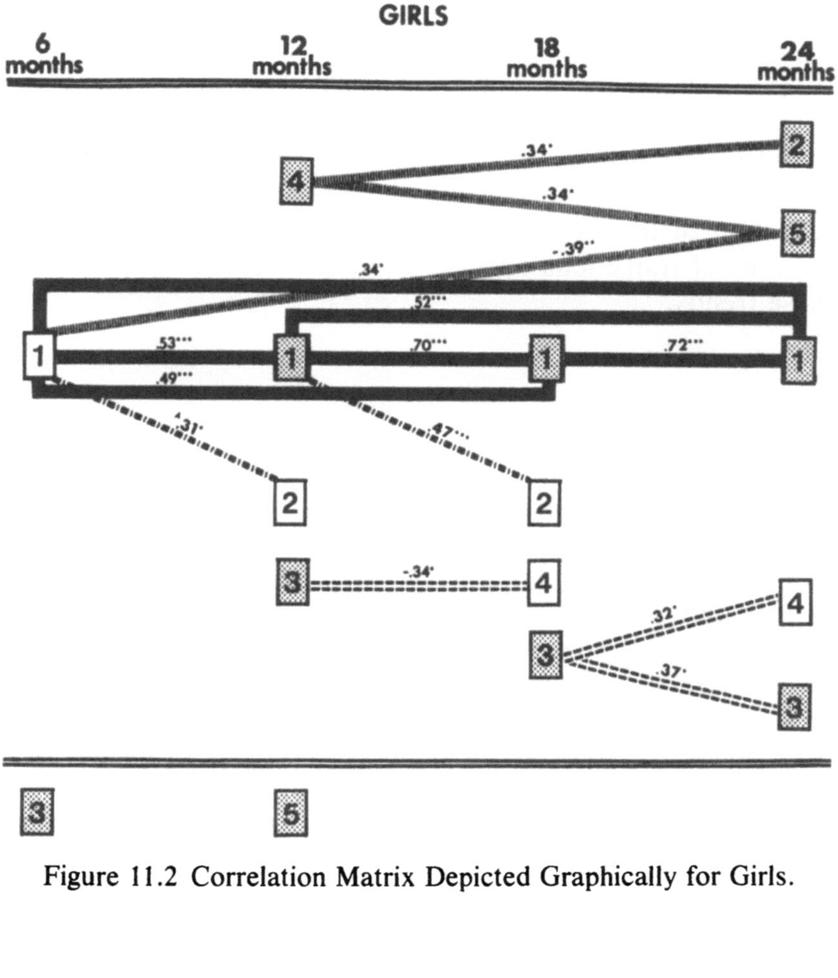

Figure 11.2 Correlation Matrix Depicted Graphically for Girls.

the fact that smaller components at 6 and 12 months did predict later IQ provokes the hypothesis that there may be other important developmental transitions that are not clearly reflected by the Gesell items (or perhaps by other infant tests).

A third point is that, although the component structure at any age in infancy was similar for males and females, the two sexes were almost totally different in the pattern of relationships across the infancy period, except for the main trend. This observation highlights the importance of the main trend in infant development but also indicates that the sexes may follow some distinctly different paths in the course of early mental development. For example, not one of the males' 12 significant cross-age correlations among smaller components is between the same pair of components represented in the 8 cross-age relationships for females.

Fourth, figures 11.1 and 11.2 suggest that the important developmental aspects during infancy are somewhat more concentrated in the main trend for girls and more fractionated and dispersed among other behavioral characteristics for boys. One reflection of this is the more complicated nature of the boys' patterns of transitions and the more cross-related character of these trends.

Interpretation

Table 11.2 presents the items having loadings of .4 or greater for each component in the main trend.

The items loading on the main developmental trend at 6 months appear to incorporate visually guided manipulation of objects and gross and fine motor behavior. However, there is another more subtle and quite provocative interpretation that links several of the fine motor and manipulation items. Many of these behaviors involve the manipulation of objects that yield perceptual contingencies behavior that has been called "the game" (Watson 1972), or involve conjugate reinforcement (Rovee & Rovee 1969). For example, the items "reaches for dangling ring," "lifts inverted cup," "bangs spoon on table," "splashes in tub," "conscious of fallen objects," and "pats table" all describe manipulation that produces a rather clear contingent perceptual consequence. The behaviors on this component are quite reminiscent of Piaget's (1952) secondary circular response in which the child repeatedly executes a simple behavior that produces an obvious perceptual consequence. Piaget observed this behavior and related activities between 3 and 8 months of life.

At 12 months, the items composing the main developmental trend still involve gross and fine motor skills, but the items reflecting visually guided manipulation and production of perceptual consequences seen at 6 months have been replaced by items requiring the imitation of fine motor behavior and the learning of rudimentary social skills. Many items on infant tests appear to reflect simple fine motor and prehensile skills. However, in many cases the examiner demonstrates the behavior and then waits for the child to imitate it. While a certain amount of fine motor skill is required to execute the behavior, passage of the item is equally dependent on the child's propensity to imitate the examiner. Consequently, the items "rings bell in imitation," "imitates rattle of spoon in cup," "builds tower of two to three cubes," "puts cube in cup," "performance box, rod in hole, (see table 11.2)" and "scribbles in imitation" all require the child to imitate the examiner.

Also loading on this component are several diverse behaviors that seem to reflect the learning of social behavior and simple verbal skills ("waves bye-bye," "says three to five words," "says bye-bye or hello," "plays peek or pat-a-cake"). The presence of these social-verbal behaviors on the same component with the imitation of fine motor behavior suggests that these are related behaviors, perhaps tied together in a social context. It seems reasonable that the child who develops the tendency to imitate probably imitates fine motor behavior first and later vocal-verbal skills in social contexts (e.g., saying hello or goodbye).

Piaget (1951) has already seen the shift in emphasis from the production of perceptual consequences to imitation as being an important dynamic transition in the early development of sen-

Table 11.2 Items, Loadings, and Correlations with Childhood IQ for the Main Trend of Developmental Transitions

6 months		*12 months*		*18 months*		*24 months*	
Component 1	Loading	Component 1	Loading	Component 1	Loading	Component 1	Loading
Reaches for dangling ring (5)	.66	Stands (3)	.63	Pictures, names several (4)	.72	Pictures, names five	.75
Exploratory manipulations of spoon, cup, saucer	.62	Walks (4)	.60	Pictures, points to several (3)	.72	Pictures, points at several (3)	.73
Regards and accepts cube (3)	.62	Takes third cube without dropping	.55	Repeats things said	.64	Speaks in sentences	.66
Lifts inverted cup, secures cube (3)	.60	Waves bye-bye	.54	Says five or more words	.60	Tells name (3)	.62
Inhibits head and one hand	.60	Rings bell in imitation	.54	Points to parts of body (3)	.59	Tells experiences	.59
Reaches directly for spoon	.58	Imitates rattle of spoon in cup	.49	Requests things at table (3)	.56	Names watch, many views (4)	.53
Sits with support, alone (3)	.56	Creeps, climbs (3)	.48	Names watch, 4th view	.52	Listens to stories with pictures	.53
Regards and secures pellet (4)	.56	Says 3 to 5 words (4)	.48	Uses two or more words together	.47	Drawing, imitates simple patterns (6)	.52
Plays with objects	.54	Builds tower of two–three cubes (3)	.47	Scribbles in imitation	.44	Uses pronouns, past, plural	.52
Bangs spoon on table	.52	Puts cube in cup (4)	.46	Throws ball in box	.43	Asks for things at table by name	.51
Purposeful reaction to paper (3)	.47	Says bye-bye or hello	.45			Names five familiar objects	.51
Splashes in tub	.45	Performance box, rod in hole	.44			Uses color names	.48
Shows consciousness of strangers	.42	Scribbles in imitation	.43			Knows prepositions (4)	.47
Conscious of fallen object (3)	.42	Tries to put on shoes	.42			Puts cube in cup, plate, box	.44
Makes stepping movements	.42	Unwraps cube	.40			Bowel control	.41
Pats table	.40	Plays peek or pat-a-cake	.40				

	Correlations with childhood IQ				
Males		S-B—3½ years: 28[a]	W-B—13 years: V: .23	S-B—3½ years: .42[c]	WISC—11 years: V: .46[b]
		6 years: .21	P: .41[b]	6 years: .38[a]	P: .28
		10 years: .20	T: .35[a]	10 years: 26	T: .42[a]
					W-B—13 years: V: .34[a]
					P: .36[a]
					T: .37[a]
Females	S-B—3½ years: [d].49[c]	S-B—3½ years: .49[c]	WISC—7 years: V: .43[a]	S-B—3½ years: .69[c]	WISC—7 years: V: .43[a]
	6 years: .46[c]	6 years: .51[c]	P: .20	6 years: .59[c]	P: .36
	10 years: .42[c]	10 years: .43[b]	T: .37[a]	10 years: .41[b]	T: .46[a]
			WISC—11 years: V: .46[b]		WISC—11 years: V: .56[c]
			P: .36[a]		P: .17
			T: .44[a]		T: .42[a]

NOTE.—See text for explanation of table.
[a] $p < .05$ for tests of the significance of a correlation.
[b] $p < .01$ for tests of the significance of a correlation.
[c] $p < .001$ for tests of the significance of a correlation.
[d] $p < .05$ for tests of sex differences for these correlations.

sorimotor intelligence. This begins as "pseudoimitation, the child. . . apparently using the imitative schema to prolong a spectacle because it corresponds to what the child is already doing [Hunt 1961, p. 133]." Later, when conceptions of object permanence, space, and causality are more mature, Piaget postulates a greater differentiation between imitative accommodation and playful assimilation, with genuine imitation as the result. Finally, the child appears to imitate "for its own sake," and begins to imitate vocal and verbal productions of the parent. Thus, the transition between the production of perceptual consequences through manipulation and the imitation of fine motor and social-vocal-verbal behavior observed in the Fels data was hypothesized long ago by Piaget as a major dynamic entity in the epigenic development in the first year.

By 18 months, the main developmental trend has become pervasively verbal in character. There are three general types of items loaded on the first principal component at 18 months. The first is verbal production ("names pictures," "repeats things said," "says five or more words," "requests things at table," "names watch," "uses two or more words together"), the second involves verbal comprehension ("points to several pictures," "points to parts of body"), and the third is an extension of the imitation of verbal and motor behavior ("repeats things said," "scribbles in imitation," "throws ball in box"). The propensity to imitate fine motor behavior and verbal skills in a social context at 12 months is related to the imitation of more complex verbal behavior and skill in verbal labeling and comprehension at 18 months.

At 24 months, the main trend has an even stronger verbal character. While there is still a hint of imitation ("imitates simple drawn patterns," "puts cube in cup, plate, box"), the predominant theme features the verbal skills of production and labeling ("names five pictures," "names watch," "asks for things at table by name," "names five familiar objects," "uses color names"), comprehension ("points at several pictures," "listens to stories with pictures"), and fluent verbal production and grammatical maturity ("speaks in sentences," "tells name," "tells experiences," "uses pronouns," "asks for things at table by name," "knows prepositions").

Although one must always be vigilant about overgeneralizations from such data and analyses, these results do provoke some hypotheses regarding the ontogeny of behavior in infancy. It is reasonable to speculate that the child who precociously develops the propensity to manipulate objects and appreciate their contingent perceptual consequences may soon apply this same strategy to the less consistent contingencies of social situations. A natural outgrowth of reciprocal social behavior is imitation, perhaps the parent imitating the child first and then the child imitating the parent. Early imitation will likely involve gross and fine motor behavior, but with development and the presence of a verbally fluent model the imitation of rudimentary language behavior subsequently emerges. Simplistically, the main behavioral trend emphasizes asocial and then social operant learning, followed by the propensity to imitate sensorimotor and then verbal behavior. Given adequate verbal models and encouragement, it is perhaps not surprising that a trend involving such basic learning processes should undergird a major developmental trend in infancy and predict later IQ.

Summary and Conclusions

When specific skill areas were determined by subjecting Gesell items taken at 6, 12, 18, and 24 months to separate principal components analyses, the correlations of component scores across these ages as well as with childhood IQs indicated several patterns of developmental transitions. The most pronounced trend spanning the entire infancy period involved the manipulative exploration of objects that produced perceptual contingencies at 6 months, the imitation of simple fine motor and elementary verbal behavior particularly in a social context at 12 months, verbal labeling and comprehension at 18 months, and verbal fluency and grammatical maturity at 24 months. Tentatively, these data highlight the potential importance of early exploration and manipulation, especially the production of contingent perceptual and social consequences, and the role of imitation as the possible developmental mediator between exploration behavior in the first 6 months and verbal production and fluency in the second year of life. The fact that this major trend of development did not predict later IQ until 12 (females) or 18 months (males) illustrates how early behavior in infancy might form the basis out of which later childhood skills emerge without itself directly predicting those childhood performances. Parallels to the epigenic development of Piaget were illustrated.

The overriding implication of this discussion is that a simple conception of a constant and pervasive g factor is probably not tenable as a model for "mental" development, especially for the infancy period. The data are strong in their denial of simple continuity of general precocity at one age with general precocity at another age during the infancy period, and emphatic in demonstrating marked qualitative shifts in behavioral dispositions. Moreover, to label as "mental" performances at every age perpetuates the belief in a pervasive and developmentally constant intelligence. Consequently, the term mental as applied to infant behavior or tests should be abandoned in favor of some conceptually more neutral label, perhaps Piaget's "sensorimotor," "perceptual-motor," or even more specific classes of behaviors (e.g., exploration of perceptual contingencies, imitation, language). The network of transitions between skills at one age and another is likely more specific and complex than once thought, and not accurately subsumed under one general concept.

12

Infant Exploration and Play

A Window on Cognitive Development

JAY BELSKY AND ROBERT K. MOST

Children's play has been a continual focus of interest to educators and psychologists, and explanations of its meaning and importance abound (Weisler & McCall 1976). One popular interpretation is that play provides opportunities to affect and control the environment in ways that the immature organism is unable to do in other contexts (e.g., Garvey 1974; White 1959). In this regard, Bruner (1973) has argued that exploration/play provides a forum for infants to develop and practice the behavioral subroutines that are subsequently integrated into more complex behavioral sequences. In essence, this position assumes that the infant acquires through play the skills and strategies that are later employed in more goal-directed activities (Weisler & McCall 1976).

In light of the significance that play has been accorded, it is surprising that until recently infant exploration and play have not received the attention they seem to merit. With the exception of Piaget's (1952) early work, exploratory activity of the infant has been studied primarily as a means of learning about infant attentional processes and the development of attachment relations rather than as a subject worthy of consideration in its own right. Thus, by measuring the *quantity* of infant exploration/play, a great deal has been discovered about the stimulus properties (e.g., novelty, moderate complexity) of objects that attract infant interest, and about the manner in which infants employ their mothers as secure bases, but the *quality* and *style* of such activity has been largely ignored (Weisler & McCall 1976). Since Piaget (1952) has shown that the manner in which infants explore their world can serve as a "window" on cognitive development, especially with respect to the practical side of intelligence (Fein 1979), this oversight is deemed significant.

In recent years several efforts have been made to correct this past neglect of the quality of infant exploration/play (e.g., McCall 1974). Students of language, for example, intrigued by the possibility that the development of gestural/language and play behavior may be programmed by the same "deep structure," have searched for parallels in the emergence and growth of these two realms of functioning (e.g., Bates 1979; Fein 1979; Nicolich 1977). Others have viewed infant play as a means of studying developmental delay (Hill & Nicolich 1979) and the effects of early experience (Belsky 1980; Belsky, Goode, & Most 1980; Rubenstein 1967). And still others have focused upon infant exploratory activity as an area of inquiry in its own right, attempting to chart developmental changes in the manner in which children manipulate play materials, some in hopes that it would illuminate the course of early cognitive development (Fenson et al. 1976; Fenson & Ramsey 1980; Fein 1979; McCall 1974; Sinclair 1970; Zelazo 1980; Zelazo & Kearsley 1980).

When considered together, the results of all these studies highlight several interesting developmental trends. For example, McCall (1974) has found that in the last quarter of the first year of life, play involving juxtapositing objects (e.g., touching two blocks together) and utilizing a toy in a manner for which it was intended (e.g., rolling a cart across the floor) increases steadily. Expanding upon this appraisal of appropriate or functional play, Zelazo and his colleagues have suggested that such play shows a marked increase toward the end of the first year of life because of a particularly noteworthy cognitive advance: the ability to generate hypotheses regarding how the world works (Fenson et al 1976; Zelazo 1980; Zelazo & Kearsley 1980). And indeed, these researchers find that such functional activity shows a curvilinear pattern between 9 and 18 months which increases precipitously only to decrease eventually in frequency of occurrence.

Such activity, it appears, is replaced as the child becomes more cognitively sophisticated and begins to engage in pretense play early in the second year (Nicolich 1977). Some debate exists at present regarding the meaning and significance of early pretend acts, which first are directed toward self (e.g., child pretends to comb his own hair with toy brush), and are only later extended to external agents (e.g., child pretends to comb doll's hair) (Fenson & Ramsey 1980; Overton & Jackson 1973; Watson & Fischer 1977). While Bates (1979) and others contend that such behavior presupposes the presence of the symbolic function—a critical achievement in early cognitive development—others regard instances of play substitution (e.g., using a stick as if it were a comb) as necessary for the appraisal of symbolic skill (Vygotsky 1967; see also Fein 1979). The argument of these latter theorists is that the relationship between the symbol and what it represents must be arbitrary to be truly symbolic, in much the same way that the correspondence between the sound of a word and its meaning is arbitrary. Thus, pretending to drink from a miniature cup, or even an empty cup, would not be true evidence of symbolic behavior, though pretending to drink from a sea shell (which has been substituted for a cup) would be. The problem with this analysis, Fein (1979) has shown, is that even early substitutions in infant pretend play cannot be considered truly arbitrary, as some objects (e.g., a stick) are more likely to serve as substitutes than are others (e.g., a ball) because of their physical similarity to the object being represented (e.g., a comb). What seems to be at issue, then, is the criteria for assessing the presence of the symbolic function in early play.

Whatever definition is adopted, there is strong agreement that play becomes increasingly sophisticated with development. Simple acts of pretend play are incorporated into elaborate sequences (e.g., feed the doll and then wipe its mouth) in much the same way, possibly, as words are strung together to make early sentences (Nicolich 1977; Bates 1979). And acts of substitution become embedded in such sequences in elaborate ways, underscoring the increasing decontextualization of early play behavior (Bates 1979; Fein 1979).

This description of play development, derived from several related studies, was drawn upon to detail a 12-step developmental sequence of infant exploration/play (see list below). To determine the validity of this developmental progression from undifferentiated exploration through decontextualized pretense play, a descriptive study of infant free play behavior was conducted, using normal infants between 7½ and 21 months of age. It was predicted that the 12-step sequence outlined below would satisfy requirements of scalability and reproducibility when investigated cross-sectionally. Moreover, it was predicted that the frequency of mouthing and simple manipulation would decrease linearly across the age span studied, while all categories of pretense play would increase linearly in frequency of occurrence. Since relational, functional relational, and enactive naming were considered to be transitional forms of manipulative activity linking early, undifferentiated exploratory behavior with later, more cognitively sophisticated pretense play, curvilinear functions were expected. Instances of these categories of exploration were hypothesized to occur at low frequencies in the last quarter of the first year, then increase to a peak in the early part of the second year, before decreasing in incidence by the second half of the second year.

Hypothesized Sequence of Development of Exploration/Play

1. Mouthing—indiscriminate mouthing of materials (e.g., mouthing peg, sea shell, etc.).
2. Simple Manipulation—visually guided manipulation lasting at least 5 seconds in duration that cannot be coded in any other category (e.g., turning over an object, touching and looking at an object, but excluding indiscriminate banging and shaking).
3. Functional—visually guided manipulation which is particularly appropriate for a certain object and involves the extraction of some unique piece of information (e.g., turn dial on toy phone,

squeeze piece of foam rubber, flip antenna of Buzy Bee, spin wheels on cart, roll cart on wheels).

4. Relational—bring together and integrate two or more materials in an "inappropriate" manner, i.e., a manner not initially intended by the manufacturer (e.g., set cradle on phone, touch spoon to stick).

5. Functional Relational—bring together and integrate two objects in an "appropriate" manner, i.e., in a manner intended by the manufacturer (e.g., set cup on saucer, place peg in hole of pegboard, mount spool on shaft of cart).

6. Enactive Naming—approximate pretense activity but without confirming evidence of actual pretend behavior (e.g., touch cup to lip without drinking sounds, tilt head back, or tip cup; raise phone receiver in proximity of ear but without talking sounds; touch brush to doll's hair but without brushing motions).

7. Pretend Self—pretense behavior directed toward self in which pretending is apparent (e.g., raise cup to lip, tip cup or make drinking sounds or tilt head; stroke own hair with miniature brush; raise phone receiver to ear and vocalize).

8. Pretend External—pretense behavior directed away from child toward other (e.g., feed doll with spoon, bottle, or cup; brush doll's hair, push car on floor and make car noise).

9. Substitution—a "meaningless" object is given meaning during a pretense act by using it in a creative or imaginative manner (e.g., drink from seashell, feed doll with stick as "bottle") or an object is used in a pretense act in a way that differs from how it was already employed by the child (e.g., hairbrush is used to brush teeth after child had already used it as a hairbrush on self or other).

10. Sequence Pretend—child repeats single pretense act with minor variation (e.g., drink from bottle, give doll drink; pour into cup, pour into plate) or child links together different pretend schemes (e.g., stir in cup, then drink; put doll in cradle, then kiss goodnight).

11. Sequence Pretend Substitution—same as Sequence Pretend but child employs an object substitution within sequence (e.g., put doll in cradle, cover with green felt piece as "blanket," feed self with spoon and then with stick).

12. Double Substitution—pretense play in which two materials are transformed, within a single act, into something they are not in reality (e.g., treat peg as doll and piece of green felt as blanket and cover peg with felt and say "night-night, treat stick as person and sea shell as cup and give stick a drink).

Method

Subjects

Forty infants between 7½ and 21 months of age served as subjects of this study, with 4 children in each of 10 evenly spaced age groups: 7½, 9, 10½, 12, 13½, 15, 16½, 18, 19½, and 21 months.

Procedure

The mother and baby were visited at home and in a quiet and isolated part of the home a set of "warm-up" toys were placed on the floor for the child to play with. While one visitor practiced narrating a description of the baby's activity into a tape recorder, the other visitor engaged the mother in conversation. The intent here was to create a comfortable situation, representative of something that might occur in the baby's everyday life—neighbors visiting and talking with the mother while the child played on the floor nearby.

Once the child was judged to be at ease, another set of toys were set out in a standard manner while the mother distracted the child with a small bell given to her for that purpose. (Toy Set One: miniature baby bottle; spoon; hair brush; 2 tea cups, 2 saucers, and a teapot; female baby doll; 4 brightly colored cylindrical sticks; sea shell; cube of foam rubber; 2 wooden clothes pins; wooden rattle; and a carnival-colored flat-bed cart on wheels, with four replaceable spools that mounted on the shafts on the cart.) At a signal, the mother set the child down on the floor and for 15 minutes the child was free to play. After 15 minutes—or earlier if the child's interest waned and could not be refocused—the mother was again given the bell to distract the child and the first set of toys was picked up and replaced by a second set of toys. (Toy Set Two: miniature baby bottle, baby, car and crib; sea shell; male baby doll; irregular-shaped piece of green felt; Fischer-Price Queen Buzy Bee and Chatter-Telephone; a home-made, large-peg pegboard; and three loose plastic "donuts".) For another 15 minutes the child was free to play with the materials provided.

Throughout the play sessions, one visitor conversed with the mother while the other narrated a description of the child's activities into a tape recorder. The mother was instructed to respond to the child's bids but not to elaborate or initiate interaction or provide the child with suggestions or directions regarding what could be done with the play materials.

The play narratives were transcribed by the observer within a few days of their recording, and then coded by other persons blind not only to the purpose of the study but also to the gender and age of the infants. Following transcriptions, the coders scored the narratives, which were divided into 10-second intervals, in terms of the highest level of play observed within a given time-sampling period. (The levels of play are defined and illustrated in the list on page 112). Since all infants did not engage the play materials for the entire 30-minute play period, it was necessary to prorate all scores in terms of a standard play period to permit comparisons between age groups. Thirty minutes was selected as the length of this standard session.

Results

Two analyses were undertaken to determine (1) if the 12-step sequence detailed in the list satisfied standard criterion of a unidimensional and cumulative scale and (2) to examine developmental changes in the frequency of 10 of the 12 play categories coded.

Individual Performance: Scalar Analysis

To determine if lower levels of play were required before higher levels could be displayed, the performance of each child was examined in terms of the levels of play that s/he showed at least one qualifying instance of. Across the entire sample, the validity and scalability of this play sequence was assessed via

Guttman scalar analysis, which tests whether later steps in the sequence are dependent upon the prior steps in the sequence; that is, for example, whether the children who show level six behavior also show levels one through five. The results of this analysis confirmed the prediction that lower levels appear before higher levels. For the 12-step sequence, the coefficient of reproducibility was .95 and that of scalability equaled .77. Thus, this scale satisfies the criteria of reproducibility (by being above .9) and scalability (by being above .6) and can be considered valid as well as unidimensional and cumulative (Nie et al. 1975).

Most of the "errors" in the hypothesized developmental sequence involved children demonstrating the ability to engage in pretense play but not showing that kind of play considered to serve as a transition from exploration to play, namely, enactive naming. These "errors" suggest that such approximations of pretend play may disappear from some children's repertoires as they successfully master more competent play routines. The same argument can be applied to that category which showed the next most frequent errors, mouthing. Infants undoubtedly grow out of the practice of relying on their mouths as tools for exploration, and we find that some infants evidence higher levels of exploration without displaying this hypothesized lowest level of object manipulation.

Group Performance: Means Analysis

To further examine developmental change in free play behavior, the number of periods in which each category of play was the highest level of play coded was subjected to a one-way analysis in variance, age being the single factor. Only 10 dependent measures were subjected to analysis, since scores on the two highest levels of play—sequence substitution and double substitution—were too small to merit analysis. These data were not discarded, however. Scores for sequence substitution were added to sequence pretend, and those from double substitution to the category substitution. Given the large number of zero scores as age-group means on some of the higher levels of play, many of the dependent variables violated assumptions of homogeneity of variance across comparison groups. Whenever this was the case, the Welch procedure was employed, since it uses heterogeneous variance estimates to calculate the F ratio (Kohr & Games 1974).

The results of these analyses revealed three general trends which are displayed in graphic form in figure 12.1. First, the frequency of mouthing and simple manipulation declined linearly across the 10 age groups, even though simple manipulation remained the most frequent kind of activity at each age period studied. Second, all types of pretend play increased linearly, with simple pretend acts (i.e., pretend self and pretend external) first appearing at 12 months of age. Finally, the hypothesized transitional categories of exploration evidenced statistically significant curvilinear trends. Scores on the measures relational, functional relational, and enacting naming started very low, then increased to a peak before declining somewhat, though never to their initially low levels.

Closer inspection of the means of the individual categories of play revealed that relational play acts were first observed earlier (7½ months) and peaked sooner (13½ months) than the next category in the hypothesized developmental sequence—functional relational (which onset at 9 months and peaked at 15 months). This result is sensible enough, as it is only logical that infants develop the capacity to relate two unrelated materials prior to discovering appropriate relationships between playthings. It is also reasonable that activity which involves making appropriate and inappropriate relationships between materials should precede pretense play, since almost all instances of pretense play involve appropriate relationships. And this is indeed what was found. Thus, for example, before a child could pretend to drink from a cup, which involved relating a cup to one's mouth, s/he would need to have the ability to generally relate materials, first in an "inappropriate" manner (relational) and then in an "appropriate" manner (functional relational).

Full-fledged pretense play did not become evident in this sample until infants were one year of age and was preceded by approximations of pretend activity. In this regard, it is interesting

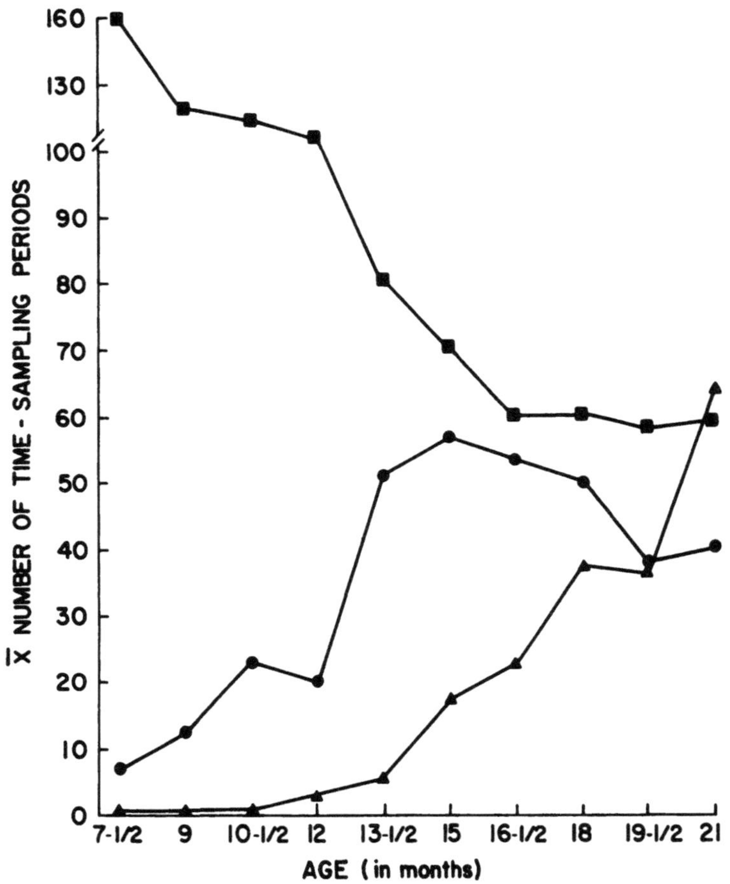

Figure 12.1 Developmental Trends in Infant Free Play Behavior

■ Undifferentiated Exploration = mouthing + simple manipulation.
● Transitional Play = relational + functional relational + enactive naming.
▲ Decontextualized Pretense Play = pretend self + pretend external + substitution + sequence pretend + sequence substitution.

to note that enactive naming increased precipitously between 9 and 10½ months, just before any instances of pretense play directed toward self were observed (at 12 months). Also of interest is the step-like fashion by which the other types of pretend occurred. While pretend self was first observed at 12 months, and then only very infrequently, instances of pretend external, sequence pretend, and substitution did not occur until 13½ months, at which point pretend other increased in frequency at a slightly faster rate than did sequence pretend, which itself increased in frequency at a slightly faster rate than substitution play.

Discussion

In its earliest form, infant exploratory behavior is seen to be undifferentiated (mouthing, simple manipulation, juxtaposing), that is, not molded to the specific nature of the object manipulated (Uzgiris 1976). In essence, "the object is what I do" during this period (McCall, Eichorn & Hogarty 1977, p. 64). In time, such exploration is modified so that the child's actions become more tailored to fit the specific features of the object (functional, functional relational). The infant seems to be guided by the question "what is this and what can it do" (Weisler & McCall 1976, p. 493). Eventually, activity with objects moves beyond the discovery of properties to the employment of preexisting knowledge in manipulating them (pretend play). We might say the child is no longer just exploring, but also playing, since behavior and behavior sequences become organism-dominated rather than stimulus dominated: "What can I do with the object" (Weisler & McCall 1976, p. 494).

Consideration of the higher levels of play detailed in the list and investigated in this report also indicates that manipulative activity becomes "decontextualized" with development (Bates 1979). That is, the "meanings represented in play become increasingly detached from particular and immediately present situations, persons, and objects" (Fein 1979, pp. 2–3). Thus, at first the child requires a real cup filled with real liquid to engage in drinking behavior, but later a miniature replica of a cup or a real though empty cup can elicit the same behavior (pretend self, pretend external). Still later, the child develops the capacity to imbue a seemingly meaningless object with meaning and thus, for example, turns a sea shell into an object from which s/he can pretend to drink (substitution). Eventually, such pretense acts are coordinated in sequences in which planning and anticipation seem to guide activity.

In summary, the results of this study provide empirical support for a developmental sequence of early exploration/play which was pieced together on the bases of select findings in the literature (e.g., McCall 1974; Fenson et al. 1976; Nicolich 1977) and the recent attempts by Uzgiris (1976) and McCall et al. (1977) to theoretically refine Piagetian analyses of infant sensorimotor development. In our data, we found that knowledge of object properties initially appear limited, with the infant's repertoire of schemes being applied indiscriminately to objects. In the course of development, however, these schemes were applied more discriminately to objects in accord with their diverse features. Eventually, conceptual relationships were drawn between objects, as the infants came to know the world apart from their own actions. Indeed, actions became coordinated by internal compensations rather than by mere trial and error, and play behavior became increasingly decontextualized and planned.

13

Early Communication and Language Development

SUSAN SPIEKER

The problem of how the young child learns language has been a major focus of theoretical and empirical inquiry within disciplines as diverse as psychology, linguistics, and anthropology. Theories explaining the process of language acquisition have ranged from environmentalistic explanations that infant babbles are shaped into speech by stimulus-response learning principles, to nativistic postulations that children are innately endowed with mental structures that contain a set of potential theories about language. Until the early 1970s, most efforts to study language acquisition focused upon children who already had language and were speaking two or more words. Investigators, influenced by Piaget's theory of sensorimotor development in infancy and by descriptions of early mother-infant interactions, then began to examine the communicative behavior of younger infants in order to discover the roots of language acquisition.

One consequence of this relatively recent focus on prelinguistic communications is that we have generated richer, though still limited, theories of the language learning process. By integrating behavioral, biological, cognitive, and social approaches to the study of language, scientists have observed some fascinating features of preverbal communicative behavior and have developed some hypotheses regarding the continuity between early social-cognitive activity and the beginnings of speech. In this paper, the preverbal period of infancy and its relation to language learning are discussed. We will consider three phases of communicative development—very early social exchanges, sensorimotor communication, and one-word utterances—before drawing some general conclusions.

Very Early Social Exchanges

Although it is common knowledge that words are not meaningful to tiny babies, young infants can respond to speech sounds and to the rhythms of spoken language. For example, one-day-old infants have been observed to move in rhythm to the acoustic boundaries of speech (as revealed by high speed photography), and neonates can sustain such synchronized movement of several body parts for sequences of over 100 words (Condon & Sander 1974). By at least one month of age, infants can discriminate between phonemes (the acoustic building blocks of language), such as "pa" and "ba," in much the same way as adults do (Eimas et al. 1971). Moreover, by the end of the first month, as many parents have noted, infants discriminate the human voice from other sounds and can be quieted by soft, high pitched talking. Theorists have used findings such as these to argue that human babies are never truly "prelinguistic" (Kaplan & Kaplan 1971), but are predisposed to acquire the ability to talk.

Another fact of human infancy that appears to be in the best interest of language acquisition is the long period of helplessness during which children are dependent on caregivers for survival; this dependency results in an affectional bond and qualities of caregiver-infant interaction which provide important experiences for learning about communication. For example, before they use words, and even before it can be claimed that they communicate intentionally, children are active partners in two-way social exchanges—what some researchers have termed "proto-conversations" (Bateson 1975). Proto-conversations have been observed between mothers and infants as young as seven weeks. These interactive, sequences are characterized by mutual eye gazing, face-to-face orientation, patterns of turn-taking (e.g., "you act, then I act"), variations in vocal intonation, and obvious mutual pleasure (Bateson 1975; Stern 1977).

There are several hypotheses explaining why participation in this kind of mutual engagement in the first months of life may be important to language development, and some of these ideas are controversial, particularly those that are efforts to prove that language results from, or is directly caused by, these early social exchanges. The first notion to be considered is that turn-taking exchanges between mothers and babies teach children their roles as partners in conversations. Snow (1977) found support for this claim in observations of mothers and infants between the ages of 3 and 18 months. Consider the following typical "conversation" between a mother and her 3-month-old:

Mother	Baby
	Smiles
Oh, what a nice little smile! Yes, isn't that pretty? There now. There's a nice little smile.	
	Burps
What a nice wind as well! Yes, that's better, isn't it? Yes Yes	
	Vocalizes
Yes! There's a nice noise.	

Note how in this exchange the baby's smiles, burps, and coos are responded to by the mother as "turns" in the conversation, thereby stimulating an appropriate response from her. Indeed, mothers often respond to such behaviors *as if* they were intended to communicate. However, even when babies do not take their turn, which can happen if they are inactive, mothers frequently "fill in" for the child. Thus, they may play the roles of both participants or behave as if the child's nonresponse is in fact a reply:

Mother	Baby
	(feeding from bottle)
Are you finished? Yes? (removing the bottle) Well, was that nice? Good, I'm glad.	

Others have looked at the infant-caregiver as a single communicative unit and, instead of focusing on "conversations," have emphasized the structure of the joint-action in caregiver-infant play routines. For example, Bruner (1977) studied the development of the game of "give-and-take" between caregivers and their 3- to 15-month-old infants with the hope of discovering that the structure of grammar emerges from the structure of these play routines. On the basis of this work, it appears that both "conversations" and play routines show similar developmental changes as the infant matures. In conversations like the ones above, the caregiver initially "fills in" for the baby's turn in the exchange. Similarly, in "give-and-take" games, the caregiver also assumes control of the exchange. Thus, the caregiver "offers" the object to the 3-month-old, and usually thrusts it into the baby's hand; the routine terminates when the baby drops the object.

By 6 months, this game has clearly become a process of the caregiver offering and the infant taking. Indeed, as the infant matures, the caregiver adds complexity and interest by offering a choice of two objects or by getting the baby to really reach for the desired object. In conversations at this age, the caregiver still carries much of the structure of the exchange, but the baby is a more active participant. As in the development of social games, the caregiver expects more of the infant during the exchange and will respond to only high quality babbles and no longer to every fret and look.

By 12 months, it is clear that the game is no longer one-sided, as babies both "give" and "take." Not only do infants at this age enjoy the task of giving and taking objects for its own sake, but they seem to understand that the game involves reciprocal roles—the Giver and the Taker. By the end of the first year, babies are also more reliably initiating turns in vocal conversations. They may be saying some words or word-like babbles, and caregivers respond as if these utterances were meaningful.

Mother	Baby
	abaabaa
Baba	
Yes, that's you, what you are.	

While proto-conversations and give-and-take games represent shared activities commonly enjoyed by preverbal infants and adults, it is not completely clear how such joint activities contribute to language development. Snow (1977) emphasizes the social turn-taking involved in these activities, and suggests that infants are learning that communication involves rules of conversation, such as "we both take turns being the Speaker and the Listener." Bruner (1977) would like to show that the structure of joint activities actually enables children to learn grammar. First, children learn the concepts, or roles, of Agent (mother), Action (give), Object (ball), Recipient (baby) on the sensorimotor level (i.e., in games), and later on, words are substituted in these action slots, so that grammatical rules are extensions of action rules.

As suggested above, theories such as these have been questioned, as it may be that systems of action schemes are largely unrelated to formal conversation rules and grammars. If this turns out to be the case, can we still accept the notion that joint-action experiences are important for language development? Yes, because it is likely that through these exchanges children learn other important aspects of communication. For example, well-understood play routines provide a perfect context for experiencing mutually shared intents. That is, both caregivers and infants come to have the same expectations for the different roles (e.g., Giver, Taker, Speaker, Listener) in a game or conversation. In these early social contexts children also learn other taken-for-granted qualities of communication, such as intersubjectivity (the experience of two persons with shared knowledge of the world) and reciprocity (sensitivity to partner) (Ryan 1974).

The establishment of such shared meanings and intentions between infants and caregivers is important because there can be no language learning unless infants and adults share the meanings to which language labels will eventually be connected. We will explore this idea further in the following discussions of the onset of intentional communication and the first use of true words.

Sensorimotor Communication

In the latter half of the second year of life a major cognitive milestone is reached which greatly facilitates the process of effective communication—the child develops the capacity to behave intentionally. While it may be impossible to pinpoint the exact onset of such intentional competence, especially since many caregivers have been responding all along *as if* their babies were communicating intentionally (often by relying on all available situational cues, e.g., wet diaper, times since last feeding), recent work by Bates and her colleagues (Bates 1979; Bates, Camaioni, & Volterra 1975) underscore the importance of the 9- to 13-month period for the emergence of intentional communication. Some time during the last quarter of the first year of life, babies can be observed to look not only at a desired object, and possibly gesture and vocalize toward it, but also alternate glances between the object and an agent (e.g., mother) whom they desire to retrieve the object for them. A child behaving in such a way appears to understand that she can use the caregiver to obtain the object. Bates et al. (1975) have called this intentional use of human agents to achieve a nonsocial goal a "proto-imperative."

There are several ways that proto-imperatives differ from behaviors that are not clearly intentional. One of the earliest indicators is alternating eye contact between caregiver and goal. Then, once the infant has "caught on" to the notion that he can influence an adult to achieve a goal, his signals become more efficient and abbreviated, or what Bates calls "ritualized." While first the infant may reach and fuss and grasp for a bottle, looking alternately from bottle to caregiver, soon he is making a ritualized open and shut movement with his hand, perhaps paired with a special vocalization, which is another ritualized form of request. Since the infant expects that these gestures will achieve a specific effect on the adult's behavior, he will look to the adult only if the desired response is not forthcoming. Another characteristic of intentional communication is that if the first effort does not work, the infant is capable of trying a second or third strategy, as in the example below.

> C is sitting in her mother's lap, while M shows her the telephone and pretends to talk. M tries to press the receiver against C's ear and have her "speak," but C pushes the receiver back and presses it against her mother's ear. This is repeated several times. When M refuses to speak into the receiver, C bats her hand against M's knee, waits a moment longer, watches M's face, and then, uttering a sharp aspirated "ha," touches her mother's mouth (Bates et al. 1975).

Infants in the Bates (1979) study also showed rapid consolidation and elaboration in the use of "proto-declaratives," which are communicative acts in which infants use objects to elicit or maintain social interactions. A proto-declarative is first observed when an infant begins showing or giving objects, alternating eye contact between the object and the adult. The baby will continue this behavior, with some variations, until he elicits the desired response (a laugh or a comment). In only a few short weeks after it first appears, this behavior becomes an efficient and ritualized signal; the baby points clearly at objects with his hand, and makes declarative-sounding vocalizations. Eventually, most ritualized proto-declaratives and proto-imperatives are recognized by both baby and caregiver as "conventional" signals; that is, there exists a shared, agreed-upon meaning for the gestures or sounds the baby makes.

As we have seen, the emergence of conventional, intentional signalling is a major event in communicative development, for the infant can now achieve certain goals in the social world. At the same time that the infant's competence in the social world is blossoming, so is his skill in the object world. Interestingly, a number of researchers have suggested that relationships exist between the child's sensorimotor competence with objects and his or her communicative development. Consider, for example, that just-discussed competence of intentional communication. To engage in such behavior, it has been suggested that infants require a basic understanding of means-ends relations (Bates et al. 1975). Such understanding not only demarcates Piaget's Stage 5 of sensorimotor development, but is also involved in such object-related tasks as obtaining a distant object set on a cloth by pulling the cloth toward oneself. Only when such capacities are in evidence is it likely that infants will be able to use adults to achieve a goal.

In all likelihood, Stage 5 sensorimotor abilities are necessary, though not sufficient, for the emergence of intentional communication. Harding and Golinkoff (1979) report that all of the infants in their study who communicated intentionally with vocalizations and eye contact also performed at Stage 5 on two Piagetian tests of causality. However, there were other infants who also performed at the Stage 5 level who did not communicate intentionally. How did the two groups of children differ? Primarily in patterns of caregiver-infant conversation and game exchanges (Harding & Golinkoff 1980). Infants in the nonintentionally communicating group (Group 1) took fewer turns in an exchange than infants in the intentionally communicating group (Group 2). Also, the Group 1 mothers took many unsolicited turns, which means that they tended to carry both sides of the exchange. When Group 1 infants did take a turn, it was most often directed at a toy, not the mother. In other words, these infants did not act as if they understood that they could communicate with the *mother* to achieve an end related to the *toy*. Harding and Golinkoff believe that these group differences are related to the mothers' styles of interacting. Group 1 mothers tended to monopolize the turns in an exchange—as if they were continuing to use a strategy of "filling in" for their babies that had been more appropriate at 7 months. They also seemed to "miss" instances of infant eye contact and vocalizations that could have been responded to as communicative initiations.

We have seen that intentional communication emerges before speech and can be influenced by early experiences. The next milestone in communicative development is the use of words.

How do children learn that words can refer to, or stand for, meanings that they may already understand? What kinds of experiences influence the words that children learn first?

Single Word Utterances

Certain comments we have made about the origins of intentional communication also apply to the beginnings of true speech. There is no clear boundary marking the advent of intentional communication; it evolves gradually in the course of social games and conversations between caregivers and infants. Once intentional communication is observed, its form develops rapidly into stable, conventional signals. It seems that the transition to word use, or true symbolic communication, is also a gradual process. However, once children catch onto the word game, at around 12 months, they start to build vocabularies at a great rate. Indeed, they may spend the next six months or so learning many new words before they make the next big advance by combining words into sentences.

The children that Bates (1979) observed between the ages of 9 and 13 months went through both of the exciting changes in communicative behavior described above. Bates reports that while the children were acquiring a stable group of conventional communicative gestures, they were also making the discovery that "things have names." Names seemed to emerge by a process of "decontextualization." This means that at first the words were tied to specific routines or situations and occur only "in context." Later they came to stand for and represent objects or events that were not immediately present. The fact that first words are context bound and only gradually become truly symbolic is a clue to understanding how children learn their first words and why some children have different styles of word acquisition.

One obvious way that children learn words is from caregivers, who all along have been talking to their infants about objects and events in their immediate environment. As we have seen, caregivers comment on the child's focus of attention or direct the child's attention and then comment. Because children speaking only one word at a time still operate at the sensorimotor stage of cognitive development, they rely on cues in the "here and now" to provide the presupposed information (knowledge shared by speaker and listener) that enables infants and caregivers to understand each other. In trying to understand what their infants are saying, or in supplying names for objects and events, caregivers assume the burden of responsibility for addressing their particular infant's focus of attention at that moment. This is usually a straightforward process. Infants are attracted to, and want to name, salient, interesting objects in their world. Thus, they will learn the words for a toy or the family cat before the words for a table or chair.

This last observation was reported by Nelson (1973) and emerged from her longitudinal study of the first 50 words acquired by 18 children. She found that most of the earliest words children learn refer to objects or events that are perceived in *action* relations. Children first name things they can manipulate or have an effect on, such as toys, food, animals, and people. Nelson found that the children in her study could be divided into two groups, depending on the categories of words they actually learned.

Nelson labeled the two groups Expressive (E) and Referential (R). E children used words that were primarily personal-social, such as "bye-bye," "more," and "naughty." R children employed words that named objects, such as "doggie," "penny," and "moo" (for cow). In part, these differences seemed to reflect differences in child rearing style on the part of the mothers. R children had mothers who were object oriented and frequently named things. E children in contrast, had mothers who focused on the child and social behaviors and were frequently very directive about the child's activities.

Although all of the children learned to use language in a variety of ways, differences between the groups persisted for some time. At two years, the R children had significantly larger vocabularies and the E children occasionally used phrases and whole sentences; however, there was no difference in the mean length of an average utterance for the two groups.

The first 10-word combinations of a high referential and a high expressive child, each 16 months old, are listed below (Nelson 1977).

Child R	Child E
Daddy all gone	I do
Daddy shoe	You do
Daddy milk	I want it
Mommy bite	I don't want it
Mommy cookie	Do it
Coat on	Don't do it
Meat bite	I love you
Spoon milk	I don't know
Blanket dirt	What d'you want
Coat wet	Go away

Even without knowing the communicative context of these utterances, it seems clear that R and E children have different ideas about the function or use of language. The R child is using words primarily to label things and describe actions on things; the E child is using words to describe people and their relationships.

Conclusions

We have reviewed some empirical observations and theoretical issues concerning prelinguistic communication and language development. The starting point in the discussion was quite simple: children learn to talk in a social environment. From the first weeks of life, children learn that social interaction is pleasurable. Shared expectations and meanings are important consequences of the special relationship between children and caregivers; they constitute the first mutually understood topics in early communicative events.

The participants in caregiver-infant exchanges are not equally skilled. During the first months, caregivers carry the structure of interactions, "filling in" for the babies' turns in the exchange. As infants become more competent, caregivers support their infants' development by yielding more and more of the action and social initiative to them, while still making every effort to follow the infants' focus of attention in order to understand what they are trying to communicate.

As children begin to communicate with gestures, they also discover that "things have names." The things that children label first may be interesting objects or personal-social actions. Language learning tends to be facilitated if both infants and caregivers share a similar focus on objects or personal-social actions. It is probably of more general importance, however, that adults manage to participate in children's language learning experiences in ways that combine sensitivity to the children's "here and now," acceptance of their imperfect utterances, and stimulation appropriate to their levels of language ability.

PART IV

Socioemotional Development

Having focussed in the preceding section on cognitive-perceptual development, we consider in this section socioemotional development. Distinctions made here between these realms of psychological functioning serve heuristic purposes and do not actually reflect reality. As Sroufe argued in his article in the opening section of this volume, the infant is an integrated whole. We dissect him for analytic purposes, and these purposes are best served when we keep in mind this need for synthesis. Thus, socioemotional and cognitive development are inextricably intertwined.

Ainsworth makes this point in the first article in this section by underscoring some of the cognitive and perceptual requirements of the attachment process. Critical steps in this process, she notes, involve perceiving the cargiver, being able to discriminate her from others, and eventually coming to understand that she exists even when she is not physically present. Ainsworth also details the theoretical foundations upon which her ideas regarding the development of the child's emotional tie to its primary caregiver are founded. Bowlby's evolutionary account of attachment behavior, which emphasizes the role that actions play in ensuring species survival, is at the core of contemporary attachment theory. In addition to defining and analyzing the function of early infant-caregiver attachment, Ainsworth details the developmental process by which a full-blown, discriminating affectional tie between mother and child comes into being.

The developmental significance of this early mother-infant relationship is empirically documented in the second article in this section. Employing an experimental procedure developed by Ainsworth to assess the quality of infant-caregiver attachment, Matas et al. report the results of a study of infants categorized as securely or anxiously attached to their mothers at 18 months of age and followed up at 24 months of age. In accord with predictions derived from Bowlby and Ainsworth's theorizing, these investigators find that those infants who could employ their caregivers as a secure base from which to explore, and who positively greeted their mothers following a stressful separation experience or were comforted by her presence, displayed more skill in problem solving and were more cooperative with their mothers than infants whose attachments were classified as insecure. Sroufe and his colleagues summarize the results of longer-term follow-up studies of these same children, results which provide additional support for the attachment theory discussed in his article, above.

While the significance of early mother-infant relations has been long recognized in the study of infancy, the importance of peers has not. Indeed, early work on infant peer relations, summarized in the third article here, indicated that during the first two years of life children had little interest and skill in engaging their agemates in interaction. Eckerman, Whatley, and Krutz, in "Growth of Social Play with Peers During the Second Year of Life," set out to test whether this early impression is indeed accurate. The results they report suggest it is not. Infants, they find, beginning as early as 10 to 12 months of age, prefer to engage agemates or toys over their mothers when in a secure context, and these preferences increase through 24 months of age. Moreover, the quantity and quality of time spent interacting with peers also changes between one and two years of age. Considered together, these results suggest that peers can developmentally influence infants but, as Eckerman and her colleagues note in concluding their article, whether peers provide an influence on development distinct from that of parents and other adults remains to be determined.

Whether or not peers and adults do indeed exert distinct influences upon infant development, the final article in this section makes clear that infants distinguish between these social agents. Indeed, the ingenious experiment reported by Michael Lewis and Jean Brooks-Gunn not only demonstrates that infants respond more positively to strange children than to strange adults, but offers support for a provocative theory as to why this should be. According to these researchers, the infant employs a "self filter" to appraise the degree of threat which a strange person represents. The more the stranger is "like one," the less the stranger needs to be feared. Thus, infants tend, as Lewis and Brooks-Gunn empirically demonstrate, to respond positively to young children and to mirror images of themselves, but to display greater wariness toward older children and adults.

14

The Development of Infant-Mother Attachment

MARY D. SALTER AINSWORTH

An attachment is an affectional tie that one person forms to another specific person, binding them together in space and enduring over time. Attachment is discriminating and specific. One may be attached to more than one person, but one cannot be attached to many people. Attachment implies affects. Although the affects may be complex and may vary from time to time, positive affects predominate, and we usually think of attachment as implying affection or love.

Animals of many species are capable of forming attachments, and these perform significant functions that promote the survival of the individual or the species. Under ordinary circumstances, the infant, whether human or animal, forms his first attachment to his mother. He is not born with a ready-made attachment to her; his attachment must develop over time, although in some species it is formed more rapidly than in others.

The Concept of Attachment

The hallmark of attachment is behavior that promotes proximity to or contact with the specific figure or figures to whom the person is attached. Such proximity- and contact-promoting behaviors are termed "attachment behaviors." Included are signaling behavior (crying, smiling, vocalizing), orienting behavior such as looking, locomotions relative to another person (following, approaching), and active physical contact behavior (clambering up, embracing, clinging). These behaviors indicate attachment only when they are differentially directed to one or a few persons rather than to others. Through such behaviors a person initiates and maintains interaction with and seeks to avoid separation from an attachment figure; through them also one keeps within range of this figure while occupied with other activities and seeks protection and reassurance from it when faced with a frightening situation.

From birth onward, an infant behaves in ways that promote proximity and contact with other persons. His cries bring others to him to intervene with efforts to terminate the cry; soon his smiles attract others to come closer and to interact with him or pick him up; and he has several primitive forms of behavior through which he is more active in seeking contact and in maintaining it. Strictly speaking, these behaviors are mere precursors of attachment, and yet they are classed as attachment behaviors since they, supplemented by other behaviors that emerge later, play an important role in the development of attachment. Moreover, even after an attachment has been formed, they continue to mediate it, and they are perhaps never entirely overridden by other, more mature forms of attachment behavior.

Even after an infant has become attached, it is necessary to distinguish between "attachment" and "attachment behavior." Attachment behavior is intermittent—sometimes present, sometimes absent. The intensity of attachment behavior varies greatly according to the circumstances of the situation. Yet attachments bridge time and distance and cannot be conceived as being present or absent, or varying in intensity, even over long periods of time. We infer the existence of an attachment from a stable propensity to seek proximity to and contact with a specific figure over time and despite all these vicissitudes. This propensity may be assumed to have some kind of intraorganismic, "structural" basis. "Attachment" refers to the propensity, whereas "attachment behavior" refers to the diversity of behaviors which promote proximity, contact, and communication with the figure or figures to whom the person is or is becoming attached.

Attachment, as here defined, is a relatively new term in the developmental sciences. It was first used by Bowlby (1958) to refer to the nature of a child's tie to his mother. He also proposed a new thory, drawing on contemporary biological science, and particularly on ethology (1969), to account for the origin of this affectional bond.

Ethologically Oriented Attachment Theory

Although it would be desirable to include in this review accounts of the origins and development of social relations that have stemmed from several theoretical orientations, space limitations lead me to focus only on that of Bowlby (1969), which I have found to be highly productive in guiding research and a useful framework within which to interpret empirical findings. Although he proposed a substantial revision of the psychoanalytic view of the origins and development of the infant-mother tie, Bowlby followed Freud in his attempt to give this and all subsequent aspects of psychological development firm roots in the biological nature of man, while perceiving in contemporary biological science, and particularly in ethology, the basis of an instinct theory that would be congruent both with the main structure of psychoanalysis and with contemporary science. He has also followed ethology in viewing the origins and development of human social relations in the setting of Darwinian evolutionary theory. Bowlby's proposal is, in effect, a substantial revision and updating of psychoanalytic instinct theory.

In his preliminary statement (1958), Bowlby proposed that an infant's attachment to his mother originates in a number of species-characteristic behavior systems, relatively independent of each other at first, which emerge at different times, become organized toward the mother as the chief attachment figure, and serve to bind child to mother and mother to child. He identified five such behavioral systems as contributing to attachment: crying and smiling, which have a signaling function and which activate maternal behavior and thus bring the adult into proximity to the child; and sucking, following, and clinging, in which the infant himself takes an active role in seeking or maintaining proximity and contact. In the course of development these behavioral systems become integrated and focused on the mother and form the basis of attachment.

Biological Roots of Attachment Behavior

The keynote of Bowlby's position is that human attachment behavior has biological roots which can be comprehended only within the context of Darwinian evolutionary principles. In the course of evolution, those components of species equipment—anatomical, physiological, and behavioral—that give survival advantages to the species (or population) are transmitted through the gene pool. Species-characteristic behavior is not limited to "fixed-action" (instinctive) patterns but may also include environmentally labile (plastic) patterns. Those species whose repertory includes a large proportion of labile behaviors are better able to cope with a wide range of environmental variations and changes than those whose repertory is largely confined to stable behavior patterns. Characteristically, the young of such species, having fewer stable, fixed-action patterns and more plasticity for learning, are less competent at birth, have a longer period of infantile helplessness, and require an extended period of parental protection and care if they are to survive. In such species it is reasonable to assume that there are genetically determined biological safeguards to sustain parental care of offspring throughout the immature period, and these include not only parental-care behavior but also reciprocal behavior in the young, namely, attachment behavior.

Biological Function of Behavior Systems

The "biological function" of a behavioral system is that which gave the species (or the individual) survival advantage in the "environment of evolutionary adaptedness"—the original environment in which the species first emerged. Basing his approach on studies of primitive hunting and gathering peoples and of ground-living nonhuman primates whose habitat is similar to man's early savannah environment, Bowlby proposed that the biological function of attachment behavior (and of reciprocal maternal retrieving behavior) is to protect the infant from danger, and especially from the danger of attack by predators.

The child's attachment behavior is in equilibrium with other important behavioral systems, notably, exploratory behavior and play. Similarly, his mother's reciprocal caretaking behavior is in some kind of balance with other adult behaviors that are antithetic to maternal care. Whereas the child's attachment behavior is directed toward seeking or maintaining the degree of proximity implied in the current set-goal, his exploratory behavior is elicited by environmental stimuli, animate or inanimate, that have features of novelty, complexity, or change. Objects possessing these features elicit approach and manipulation and may draw the child away from his mother; but when he reaches the distance determined by the current set-goal of proximity, attachment behavior is usually activated and he turns back toward his mother. Thus there is balance between exploring away from and seeking proximity to the mother. At the same time, the mother's behavior shows some equilibrium between retrieving the child (thus bringing him into closer proximity) and achieving other set-goals related to her other interests and activities. The implication is, however, that if the infant strays too far or stays away too long, the mother's retrieving behavior is likely to be activated, and certainly if there is any reason for alarm she becomes concerned not merely to keep the infant within a reasonable supervisory distance but to have him close to her. And, of course, the child's set-goal may change from one of considerable distance from his mother to one of closest contact with her if he becomes alarmed or distressed.

Sequential Phases in the Development of Attachment

At least four major phases in the development of attachment may be distinguished: a phase during which social responsiveness is relatively undiscriminating; a phase of discriminating social responsiveness; a phase marked by emergence of active initiative in proximity-seeking, contact-seeking, and contact-maintaining behavior; and a final phase identified by Bowlby (1969) as one of goal-corrected partnership.

1. Phase of Undiscriminating Social Responsiveness. During this first period, which spans roughly the first two or three months of life, the infant has the capacity to orient himself to salient features of his environment, especially to people. Some of his various orienting, signaling, and active proximity- and contact-promoting behaviors are most easily terminated by other stimuli coming from humans. His orienting behaviors include visual fixation, visual tracking, listening, rooting, and postural adjustment when held. He also has some primitive behaviors—sucking and grasping—through which he actively gains or maintains contact. He has a number of special signaling behaviors—smiling, crying, and other vocalizations—that tend to activate adult behavior and have the "predictable outcome" of bringing his mother (or other care-givers) into proximity or contact with him. (Indeed, to a perceptive mother the infant's entire behavioral repertory has a signaling function.)

The infant's initial sensory equipment is remarkably efficient and capable of rapid improvement. From the beginning he has some capacity to respond differentially to different stimuli and hence to discriminate them. Furthermore, the range of stimuli to which he is most responsive includes the range commonly emanating from human adults, including visual and auditory stimuli as well as stimuli associated with feeding. But despite his innate discrimination between classes and ranges of stimuli, he does not at first discriminate between the persons presenting these stimuli.

Although "genetic bias" determines differential sensitivity from the outset, changes are rapid during these earliest months. Direct effects of differential environmental influences are clearly identifiable as well as the indirect effects these may have on maturational process.

The transition between this phase and the subsequent discriminative phase of social responsiveness is not clear-cut. Discrimination between persons is learned more rapidly through some modalities than through others. There is reason to believe that tactual-kinesthetic discrimination may come first and auditory discrimination next, but visual discrimination is unlikely to occur earlier than eight weeks of age.

2. *Phase of Discriminating Social Responsiveness.* During this phase the baby continues to orient and to signal, but he clearly discriminates between familiar figures (his mother and one or two others) and those who are relatively unfamiliar, and he is differentially responsive. Ainsworth (1967) distinguished two phases, which are here combined: one in which there is discrimination and differential responsiveness to figures close at hand, and a second in which discrimination can be made between figures at a distance. Differential smiling, vocalization, and crying emerge in the first, and differential greeting and crying when the figure leaves the room come in the second.

The end of this phase comes with the emergence of more active proximity-seeking and contact-maintaining behaviors, perhaps as early as six months of age, perhaps later, according to rearing conditions and sensorimotor development.

3. *Phase of Active Initiative in Seeking Proximity and Contact.* During this phase all the earlier attachment behaviors are still present and differential, but there is a striking increase in the baby's initiative in promoting proximity and contact. His signals are no longer merely expressive or reactive; they often are intended to evoke a response from the mother or other attachment figure. Locomotion facilitates proximity seeking, and voluntary movements of hands and arms are conspicuous now in attachment behavior. Greeting responses become more active and effective. Following, approaching, clinging, and various other active contact behaviors become significant. The median age for attaining this phase is about seven months.

Bowlby (1969) suggests that "goal-corrected" sequences of behavior emerge in this phase: sequences guided by a constant stream of feedback so that the baby alters the direction, speed, and nature of his behavior in accordance with that of the figure to whom he has become attached, and later also in accordance with a "plan." Indeed, it is in this phase that the baby is usually first described as attached. It also coincides with the period during which psychoanalytic theorists judge "true object relations" to emerge. Further, its onset coincides with Piaget's fourth stage of sensorimotor development, in which the child first begins to search for hidden objects and thus manifests the beginnings of the concept of an object as permanent despite its not being present to perception. This feature of cognitive development may index the inner structural basis for attachment.

4. *Phase of Goal-Corrected Partnership.* Although previous research into the development of attachment had dealt chiefly with the first three phases, Bowlby (1969) sketched the characteristics of a fourth phase. In the third phase, although the baby could to some extent predict his mother's movements and adjust his own to them in order to maintain the degree of proximity he currently desired, he could not understand the factors that influenced these and could not plan means to change her behavior. Gradually, however, he comes to infer something about his mother's "set-goals" and about the plans she is adopting to achieve them. Only then can he begin to attempt to alter her set-goals and plans to fit better with his own in regard to contact, proximity, and interaction. Bowlby characterizes the more complex and sophisticated relationship which ensues as a "partnership." This phase of development has been least investigated, and so it is difficult to specify even an approximate age of onset. Bowlby's best guess is that it usually does not begin until about age three, although it may occur earlier in some children. Bowlby considers as relevant Piaget's concept of "egocentrism" (1951, 1952). In his first efforts to change the set-goal of his mother's behavior, a young child is handicapped by his inability to see things from her point of view. Therefore, the reciprocity of the partnership is primitive at first and develops only gradually. Furthermore, a child may be hampered by the extent to which his mother dissembles about her set-goals and discourages him from perceiving what they are.

Certainly in this phase, and probably earlier in phase three, we have a child who is attached to his mother or principal caregiver. Once formed, this attachment is amazingly persistent, and is capable of enduring an extraordinary amount of absence, neglect, or abuse—although these adverse conditions are likely to affect both the quality of a child's attachment relationship and his subsequent personality development.

15

Continuity of Adaptation in the Second Year

The Relationship between Quality of Attachment and Later Competence

LEAH MATAS, RICHARD A. AREND, AND ALAN SROUFE

Theoretical formulations of emotional development in childhood (e.g., Erikson 1963; Escalona 1968; Loevinger 1976; Mahler 1975) and early intervention efforts rest on the assumption of continuity in adaptation. It is assumed that there is coherence in personality development over time, that early assessments predict the presence of later developmental difficulties, and that particular difficulties are linked to the quality of early adaptation in a logical manner.

This study was designed to test the power of a particular perspective on continuity in early development. Within this perspective it is assumed that despite qualitative advances in developmental level and despite dramatic changes in the behavioral repertoire, there is continuity in the quality of adaptation or the way in which behavior is organized (Sroufe 1979; Sroufe &

Waters 1977). The quality of adaptation is assessed by examining the child's functioning with respect to issues salient for the particular developmental period.

From a variety of theoretical perspectives, for example, the well-functioning or competent 12–18-month-old is one who has formed an attachment relationship which effectively supports active exploration and mastery of the inanimate and social environment. Such mastery is a central task for this age period (Ainsworth 1973; Erikson 1963; Mahler 1975; Piaget 1952). From this viewpoint, difficulty separating from the attachment figure to explore novel aspects of the environment or difficulty deriving comfort from the caregiver when distressed (and readily returning to play/exploration) are maladaptive.

Similarly, the well-functioning 2-year-old has made great strides toward autonomous functioning and further progress in the separation-individuation process (e.g., Erikson 1963, Mahler 1975). For example, in a problem-solving situation, movement toward autonomy would be indicated by flexibility, resourcefulness, and ability to use adult assistance without being overly dependent on it. The competent toddler becomes readily and eagerly involved in a task, shows pleasure in task solution, and, in the face of frustration, remains involved and examines alternative strategies before giving up all efforts at solving the problem.

From infancy to early childhood, then, the prediction is that the child with a secure, effective attachment relationship will later exhibit competent, more autonomous functioning in terms of both affective involvement and problem-solving style. Such a prediction is made both from the assumption of coherence in personal adaptation and because adaptation at the earlier developmental phase can be seen to lay the groundwork for later adaptation. The child whose early exploration of the environment is supported by a positive attachment relationship will gain not only object-mastery skills, but also a sense of effectance (see White 1959). He or she will be confident of emotional support when exploratory activities lead to stress and will experience an amplification of his/her involvement through affective sharing of mastery-play activities. The greater ability to invest oneself in the world is seen as leading to greater competence (Ainsworth & Bell 1974).

Ainsworth has provided a method for assessing attachment that is well suited to the research problem at hand (e.g., Ainsworth, Bell, & Stayton 1971; Ainsworth et al. 1978). In this system, which is based on Bowlby's (1969) ethological theory of attachment as affective bond, individual differences in the quality of attachment are explicitly defined in terms of attachment/exploration balance, use of the caregiver as a base for exploration, and ability to derive comfort from the caregiver's presence, interaction, or contact. Ainsworth's strange-situation procedure is a cumulative-stress situation which taxes the infant's capacity for coordinating adaptive response and thus represents an appropriate, broad-band assessment of competence. The emphasis is on the way in which attachment behavior is organized by the individual across contexts and with respect to other behavioral systems (Sroufe & Waters 1977). Moreover, her classification system has been shown to be highly reliable, to yield stable individual differences, and to have a variety of external correlates, including home behavior (see Ainsworth et al. [1978]; Sroufe & Waters [1977] for reviews).

Given this well-developed and validated system for assessing secure attachment as an important indication of successful adaptation in late infancy, the remaining task was to develop comparable assessments of adaptation for the early toddler period and to determine the strength of the link from early to later behavior. We elected to use a tool-using, problem-solving situation. Some of the problems were readily solved and some were well beyond the capacity of the 2-year-old, but the child's mother was available for assistance. Thus, like the Ainsworth paradigm, this situation taxed the capacity of the child for coordinating affect, cognition, and behavior, and for drawing upon personal and environmental resources. By focusing on task involvement, persistence, ability to use adult resources, and other aspects of problem-solving style, it was felt that the quality of the toddler's adaptation could be captured in this situation.

In this study infants were classified as to the quality of their attachment relationship based on 18-month strange-situation behavior. A measure of cognitive competence (Bayley Mental Developmental Scales) was administered at 23 months. Finally, at 24 months the child's play behavior and problem-solving behavior were assessed. In this latter situation, maternal support and assistance also were evaluated. While the age span studied is narrow, the period in question marks an important transition in every developmental stage theory (e.g., Erikson 1963; Mahler 1975; Piaget 1952). It marks the transition between infancy and childhood, from prerepresentational to representational thought. Moreover, it is a period in which developmental discontinuity (rapid change; failure of early assessments of developmental level to predict later assessments strongly) has been amply demonstrated (e.g., McCall 1977). Therefore, a demonstration of continuity in personal adaptation across this age span is of some significance.

Method

Subjects

The sample consisted of 25 male and 23 female white, middle-class infants and their mothers. Half of the subjects were first-born; half had at least one older sibling.

Procedure

Assessment of attachment. Eighteen-month-old infants and their mothers were observed in a standard laboratory setting. Quality of attachment was assessed using the Ainsworth paradigm (Ainsworth & Wittig 1969; Sroufe & Waters 1977). This is a cumulative-stress situation with two separations and reunions, the latter involving the infant's being left alone briefly. While there are eight specific categories, infants are classified into three main groups: securely attached (group B, approximately 70%), avoidant (group A, approximately 18%), and ambivalent (group C, approximately 12%). The classifications reflect the pattern of behavior across the eight episodes of the strange situation but are heavily determined by reunion behavior. Securely attached babies are active in seeking physical contact or interaction on reunion, and this contact is effective in terminating distress and promoting a return to absorbed play. Avoidant infants avoid the caregiver upon reunion, especially the second reunion when distress is presumed to be greater. Ambivalent babies have difficulty becoming settled upon reunion and may mix contact seeking with squirming to get down, pushing away, batting toys, and other signs of contact resistance.

Assessment of free play and cleanup. At 24 months the toddlers returned to the laboratory for a 10-minute free play period, a 6-minute cleanup period, and the problem solving tasks. Within the free play period, naturally occurring bouts of symbolic play were coded. Symbolic play bouts consisted of behaviors clearly showing pretending and imagination, such as placing a small wooden person in a tractor seat and having him "drive" around, placing the animals in the barn, or "pouring" a cup of tea and offering it to the mother. To qualify as a bout the play had to last 5 seconds or more. If the child switched his attention from its original activity, or if the original play bout was interrupted by 5 or more seconds of inactivity or inattention, this was designated as the end of the original bout and initiation of the next bout if appropriate. Further, although the mothers were requested to refrain from initiating play, if they did so, the mother-initiated instance of imaginative play was not coded as a symbolic play bout.

Following free play, the mother initiated the cleanup period. This allowed observation of the child when an ongoing, pleasant activity was interrupted. The following behaviors were coded in the cleanup task by means of frequency counts made from the videotapes: (1) oppositional behavior—child says "no" in response to mother's request or does the opposite to what he is told; and (2) angry behavior—child engages in foot stomping, hitting, whining or crying, temper tantrums, leaving the task, or physical struggles with the mother.

Assessment of problem-solving style. Following the 10-minute free play period and the 6-minute cleanup period, the subjects were presented with four problem solving tasks. The experimenter explained the problems to the mother and presented the apparatus to the child, but then withdrew to the far corner of the room. Mother was told to let the child first work on the problem independently, then to give "any help you think he/she needs." The first two problems were simple: removing a lure from a space between two closely spaced wooden panels or from a tube, using a stick. The other two problems were increasingly difficult: putting two sticks end to end in order to get a lure from a long tube and weighting down the end of a lever with a block to raise candy through a hole in a Plexiglas box. Two-year-olds cannot solve the latter task without the help of an adult.

The following rationally derived measures were scored from videotape recordings of the tool-using situation and were coded without knowledge of the attachment assessments or of play behavior. Only the final two problems were coded, the initial two problems being readily solved and viewed as warm-up tasks. For those subjects taking longer than 6 minutes to solve a given problem, the first 3½ and last 2½ minutes were coded. A number of measures were based on frequency counts (converted to percentage of maternal directives for the first four variables): (1) compliance—child complies with mother's suggestion; (2) attempted compliance—child attempts to comply with suggestion but does not fully carry it out; (3) active noncompliance—child's behavior is almost exactly contrary to mother's suggestion; (4) ignoring—child ignores mother's suggestion; (5) verbal negativism—"no" in response to mother's suggestion; (6) frustration behavior—hitting, kicking, foot stomping, scratching, or biting; (7) aggressive behavior—hitting, kicking, pushing, scratching, or biting directed at mother; (8) whining or crying; (9) help seeking—instance of seeking help from mother coded and timed; and (10) time away from task—nontask behavior, timed in seconds.

In addition, rating scales were used to assess enthusiasm (seven-point scale), positive affect (three-point scale), and negative affect (four-point scale) during problems three and four.

A high score on supportive presence involved meeting two major criteria: (1) providing a "secure base" by helping the child feel comfortable with working at the task; and (2) being involved, as manifested by the mother's attentiveness to the child and the task, as well as by several minor criteria (e.g., focusing the child on the task as needed, mood setting for a problem-solving situation, sharing in the joy of problem solution, being physically present when needed, helping the child achieve a sense of having solved the problem himself). Lower scores were given according to the number of these criteria that were not met.

A high score on quality of assistance involved meeting the major criteria of helping the child see the relationship between the actions required to solve the problem and giving the minimal assistance needed to keep the child working and directed at solving the problem without solving it for him, as well as several minor criteria (e.g., giving space initially, timing and pacing the cues, giving cues the child could understand, having control of the situation, cooperating with the child). Again, lower scores on this scale were given according to the number of criteria that were not met.

Assessment of developmental level. At 23 months the Bayley Mental Developmental Scales were administered to the first group of 37 subjects by a trained tester in another room at the Institute of Child Development. The mother remained with the child throughout the testing session.

Results

Findings Descriptive of This Sample

Sixty-two percent of the sample randomly selected for this study were classified as securely attached, which is in approximate agreement to previous findings (e.g., Ainsworth et al. 1978; Waters 1978). Including the 11 avoidant and ambivalent infants from a previous study, there were 23 securely attached, 15 avoidant, and 10 ambivalent babies.

The average developmental quotient (DQ) of the total sample was 115.25, reflecting the middle-class status of the sample. While means favored the securely attached subjects, their DQs were not significantly higher than either the avoidant or the ambivalent groups (table 15.1).

There was an average of only 1.04 instances of negativism in the approximately 12 minutes of tool using. However, in the clean-up task, which lasted 6 minutes, there was an average of 2.05 instances of negativism. This task, which interrupted 10 minutes of free play, seems to be the type of situation where more typical oppositional behavior (though rarely temper outbursts) is noted. Most interesting, the securely attached infants showed more oppositional (though less angry) behavior in the clean-up period but dramatically and significantly less during the problem solving, where compliance with the mother has a clear adaptive advantage (see table 15.1).

Attachment Classification and Symbolic Play

Means and standard deviations for each attachment group on frequency of symbolic play are found at the bottom of table 15.1. Analysis of variance and subsequent *t* tests (two-tailed) indicated that securely attached infants engaged in more imaginative, sym-

Table 15.1 Means for Dependent Variables

Measures	Group B	Group A	Group C
1. Bayley Mental Development Index	118.96	108.89	108.25
2. Percent comply	.36	.22	.20
3. Percent comply or attempt comply	.57	.39	.40
4. Percent Active noncompliance	.04	.07	.05
5. Percent ignoring	.26	.44	.46
6. Percent time away from task	.12	.24	.17
7. Number seeking help	4.48	7.60	7.80
8. Enthusiasm rating (both tools)	9.22	6.08	7.70
9. Proportion saying "no"	.22	.60	.30
10. Number showing frustration behavior	.65	2.67	1.70
11. Proportion engaging in agressive behavior	.00	.33	.10
12. Proportion crying or whining	.52	.72	.80
13. Proportion seeking help within 30 seconds	.30	.53	.60
14. Propostion = "3" on positive affect	.26	.07	.00
15. Proportion = "3" or "4" on negative affect	.13	.43	.20
16. Mother's supportive presence (two tools)	10.04	5.53	6.20
17. Mother's quality of assistance (two tools)	10.04	5.00	5.70
18. Cleanup: oppositional behavior	3.81	3.00	2.11
19. Cleanup: angry behavior	1.71	2.00	3.22
20. Bouts of symbolic play	3.40	1.35	.12

bolic play than both avoidant ($p < .02$) and ambivalent ($p < .02$) infants.

Attachment Classification and Adaptive Behavior

Analyses of variance and subsequent orthogonal linear contrasts for the continuously distributed variables (items 2–8 and 10 in table 15.1) revealed that the securely attached (group B) infants were more enthusiastic ($p < .005$) and complied with maternal requests more frequently ($p < .0001$) than non-B babies; they ignored the mother less ($p < .0001$), spent less time away from the task ($p < .06$), and exhibited fewer frustration behaviors ($p < .039$). One-tailed tests of proportions on the dichotomous or trichotomous variables indicated that infants classified as securely attached at 18 months were also higher on positive affect ($p < .01$) and lower on saying "no," crying or whining, negative affect (all $p < .05$), and engaging in aggression toward mother ($p < .01$). Since, as will be discussed below, comparisons of the securely attached infants with the avoidant subgroup are of special theoretical importance, seven measures selected a priori were also considered for these two groups separately (active noncompliance, ignoring, time away, "no," enthusiasm, positive affect, aggression). Significant differences favoring the securely attached infants (.05 and beyond) were found for each of these comparisons with the exceptions of active noncompliance and "no," which were also in the predicted direction.

Maternal variables. As table 15.1 shows, the two assessments of maternal behavior—the supportive presence and quality of assistance scales—significantly differentiated securely attached from insecurely attached infants during the tool-use problems ($p < .001$).

Discussion

White (1959) defined competence in terms of an organism's capacity to interact effectively with its environment. In attempting to adapt this definition to an understanding of competence in infancy, Ainsworth and Bell (1974) viewed an infant as competent "to the extent that he can, through his own activity, control the effect that his environment will have on him." This definition of competence characterizes the competent mother-infant pair as "an infant who is competent in his preadapted function and a mother who is competent in the reciprocal role to which the infant's behavior is preadapted."

The tasks of the present study were the redefinition of competence in terms of second-year adaptation and the demonstration of continutity between adaptive functioning in infancy and adaptive functioning at 24 months. The variables investigated at 24 months reflect a broad range of characteristics that enter into the child's interaction with his environment in both social and cognitive domains. Although the dimensions of adaptive functioning assessed at age 2 were not of central concern in the earlier developmental period, they were nevertheless predictable from the assessments of adaptive functioning at 18 months.

Subjects classified as securely attached in infancy subsequently showed a significantly greater amount of symbolic play, even though they did not differ on DQ. In the tool-using tasks they were significantly more enthusiastic, affectively positive, and persistent; they exhibited less nontask behavior, ignoring of mother, and noncompliance. Separate analyses also suggested securely attached infants to be less actively oppositional and less easily frustrated, and to exhibit less crying and negative affect.

In general, however, the two groups of infants whose insecurity in their primary attachment relationship was manifested by avoidant and ambivalent behavior at 18 months showed a poorer quality of adaptation at 2 years. All relationships were in the predicted direction, and in many cases there was virtually no overlap in the scores of securely and insecurely attached children. Support is thus provided for a developmental perspective that would predict continuity between earlier and later adaptive functioning even in the absence of behavioral isomorphism. These results are in agreement with those of Waters (1978) and those of Main (1973), who also found securely attached infants to be more socially and cognitively competent as toddlers. In each of these studies the continuity has been shown for middle-class samples where relative stability of the environment can be assumed.

The predicted continuity is perhaps most striking in the case of the avoidant babies. Whereas the maladaptation of the ambivalent babies is readily apparent from their inordinate intolerance of separation, their difficulty, in being comforted; and their poverty of exploration, the maladaptation of the avoidant babies in the strange situation is not self-evident. In the 18-month strange situation these avoidant babies spent a lot of time with the toys, engaged the stranger, tended to cry only when left alone, and stopped crying when the stranger returned prior to reunion with the mother. They did not tantrum and were not petulant. Indeed, to some they would appear precociously independent. But the absence of greeting and the failure to initiate contact or interaction upon reunion with the caregiver, especially subsequent to a distress experience, suggested maladaptation. Interference with expectable attachment behavior by an underlying affective process (anger or anxiety), or perhaps, more parsimoniously, an approach-avoidance conflict, was inferred (see Main [1977] for a more extensive discussion). It is on the basis of this inferred process, reflected in avoidant behavior, that later aggression, noncompliance, and lack of persistence and affective involvement were predicted, though this had not been the pattern of behavior observed at 18 months.

An understanding of continuity in development requires a theoretically-based appreciation for qualitative changes in development, their precursors, and their correlates. Relationships in this study were powerful. According to the theoretical position adopted here, the continuity observed is based not only on the assumption that the attachment relationship provides a secure base for exploration of the environment, but also on the organizational significance of affective dimensions of behavior (Sroufe 1979). In the second year, with the emergence of more symbolic (particularly verbal) aspects of cognitive development, one would not expect that intellectual competence and earlier exploration would be closely related or that there would be a direct relationship between quality of attachment and cognitive competence.

The dependent variables in the present study were not, therefore, primarily related to "skill"; rather, they were related to the child's style or approach to problem solving. These latter dimensions were seen as associated with the attachment relationship in that this relationship is an important aspect of infant emotional development, the secure base serving as a context within which the infant develops its first reciprocal relationship with another individual, its rudimentary sense of self, and its first sense of the emotional availability and sensitivity of others. It was expected that children whose primary attachment relationship provided a secure base, in this broader sense, would be freer to involve themselves in new objects and to invest themselves in problem solving and would not be preoccupied with gaining the mother's attention or with frustrating her efforts to help them.

Competence in the 2-Year-Old

The ability to function effectively in the face of frustration, to utilize external assistance appropriately, and to refrain from excessively self-defeating behavior are typically seen as hallmarks of ego development (Loevinger 1976). The child who is capable of such behavior is one who is beginning to develop an appropriate, realistic, and secure sense of self. "From a sense of self-control without loss of self-esteem comes a lasting sense of good will and pride" (Erikson 1963 p. 255).

The competent 2-year-old as seen in the present study is not the child who automatically complies with whatever the mother tells him/her. Rather, it is the child who shows a certain amount of noncompliance when requested to stop playing and clean up the toys, but who gradually cooperates with the mother. When, however, cooperation has clear adaptive advantage, as in the tool-using situation, these children become readily involved in the task, sharing their enthusiasm with the mother and frequently with the experimenter. They work hard, independently at first, then request help from the mother when they get stuck. They tend to cooperate, or attempt to cooperate, with many of the mother's suggestions for solving the problem.

The differing patterns of oppositional behavior across contexts illustrate the difference between the construct of secure attachment and a negative temperament construct. As toddlers, securely attached infants can be oppositional; in fact, they tended to be more so when asked to stop doing something they wanted to do. But they are not so oppositional when they need and are seeking the caregiver's help. Toddlers who were ambivalent and avoidant babies, on the other hand, despite their seemingly opposite features at 18 months (much crying and contact seeking vs. contact avoiding and little crying), are similar in showing much noncompliance during the tool-using problems.

16

Growth of Social Play with Peers During the Second Year of Life

CAROL O. ECKERMAN, JUDITH L. WHATLEY, AND STUART L. KUTZ

Scant attention has been paid to the social interactions between children under two years of age, despite the importance attached to early peer interactions by students of nonhuman primates (e.g., Harlow 1969; Hinde 1971) and despite repeated observations of human infants exchanging glances, sounds, smiles, and even toys (e.g., Bridges 1933; Bühler 1930; Vincze 1971). Our knowledge of early human sociability remains limited in large measure to child-mother interactions and to children's initial reactions to unfamiliar adults (e.g., Rheingold & Eckerman 1973; Schaffer 1971). Yet the interactions between infant peers may mirror the social development occurring through child-adult interaction; and even more important, interactions with peers may contribute in their own right to early social development.

The most comprehensive prior study of interactions between children under 2 years of age is that of Maudry and Nekula (1939), conducted in a foundling home over 30 years ago. Pairs of children 6 to 25 months of age were placed together in a playpen, usually with only a single toy, and prompted into interaction. Maudry and Nekula concluded that infants at first fail to distinguish between each other and inanimate objects (6 to 8 months), later treat each other as obstacles to play materials

(9 to 13 months), and only when approaching 2 years of age (19 to 25 months) view each other as social partners—a progression that differs markedly from that proposed for infants' interactions with adults (e.g., Schaffer 1971). Their conclusion, however, was based upon viewing institutionalized children in a single, and probably unusual, setting.

In the present study, paris of normal, home-reared children were brought together in a controlled play setting which included their mothers. The children, similar in age and unfamiliar to one another, were left free to interact with several new toys, their mothers, or one another. The goals were (1) to describe the extent and forms of interaction that the children freely engaged in with one another (2) to assess changes over the second year of life in their interactions, and (3) to compare their behavior with one another to that with their mothers and with novel inanimate objects. Such as examination of interactions among young peers is a prerequisite for reasoning about the role of peers in normal human social development.

Method

Subjects

The subjects were 60 normal, home-reared children, equally divided into three age groups—10.0 to 12.0, 16.0 to 18.0, and 22.0 to 24.0 months of age—and paired within each group on the basis of age alone.

Study Setting

The study took place in a room of moderate size (2.8 × 2.9 m), unfurnished except for a few animal pictures on the walls beyond the subjects' reach and several toys on the floor. The toys were a pulltoy with marbles enclosed in a clear plastic ball, a large plastic dump truck, and three 9-cm-square vinyl cubes decorated with pictures and litters; each toy was present in duplicate. Cushions on the floor in opposite corners along the room's length marked the mother's positions; the toys were spaced along the wall opposite the mother's positions. A one-way window behind the toys provided visual access; a microphone in the center of the ceiling, auditory access.

Procedure

Each subject and his mother were escorted to a reception room where they met the other mother and child and the female experimenter. For approximately 5 minutes the children were left free to sit on their mothers' laps or to explore the room and the few toys it contained while the experimenter instructed the mothers in their role. They were asked to talk naturally with one another, allowing their children to do as they wished; they could respond with a smile or a word or two to the children's social overtures, but they were not to initiate interaction with them or direct their activities unless intervention was necessary to prevent physical harm.

The mothers carried the subjects into the study room, placed them on the floor before the toys, and sat at their positions on the floor. The experimenter then left the room, closing the door behind her, and the 20-minute session began. At the end of the session, the experimenter obtained from the mothers information about the family and the children's prior exposure to peers.

Response Measures

An observer behind the one-way window systematically sampled each child's behavior. He focused upon one child at a time and alternated 15-second periods of observation with 15-second periods of recording. Every four observation periods, or 2 minutes, the focus shifted from one child to the other. The resulting record thus was based upon 40 observations, 20 of each child. For each observation, the observer recorded whether or not each of 21 behaviors occurred; the frequency of the behavior within the 15-second period was not recorded.

Results

Reactions to the Novel Play Setting

The subjects of all ages interacted with the toys and their peers, and they contacted their mothers little (see figure 16.1). A multivariate analysis of variance on the three measures indicated a reliable change in behavior with age, F (6, 50) = 3.42, $p < .01$. Both the frequency of interactions with the peer and contact with the toy increased reliably with age, F (2, 27) =

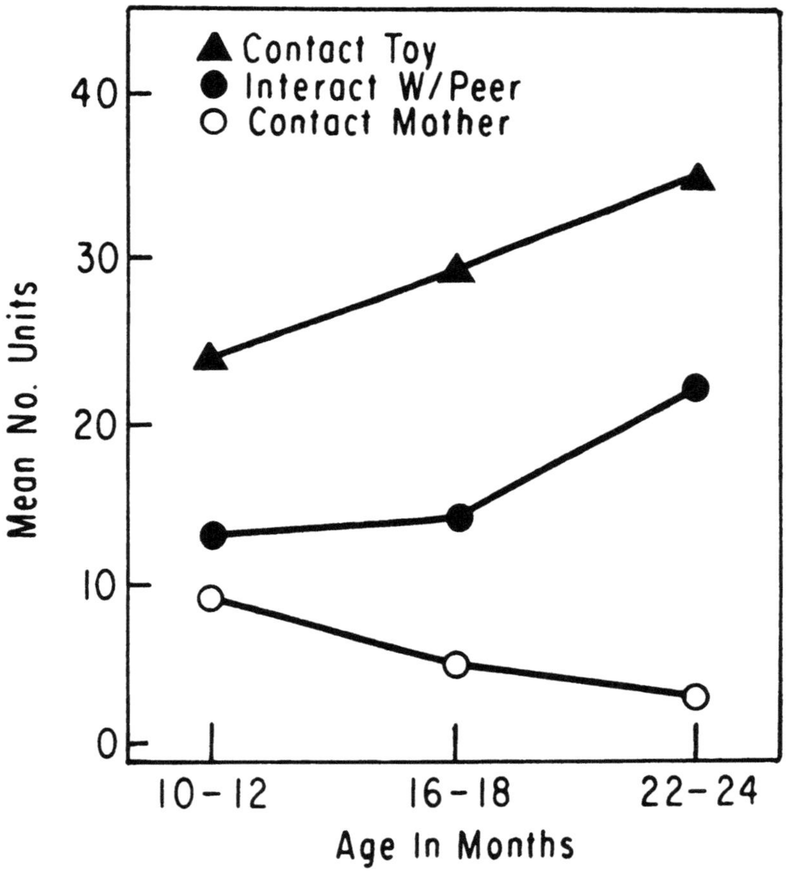

Figure 16.1. General Reaction to the Novel Play Setting.

5.90, $p < .01$; F (2, 27) = 8.38, $p < .001$; in contrast, contact with the mother decreased, F (2, 27) = 7.73, $p < .01$.

Fussing and crying occurred infrequently, during an average of only one of the 40 periods at each age; and at each age, smiling or laughing occurred more frequently (M = 2.6, 4.7, and 5.1 periods for the 10–12-, 16–18-, and 22–24-month groups, respectively). Some fussing or crying occurred in 14 pairs; smiling or laughing, in 22 pairs.

Nature of the Interactions with the Peer

The subjects attended to the peer (i.e., one or more peer-related behaviors occurred) in over 60 percent of the observations at each age. Table 16.1 summarizes the results for each peer-related behavior. A multivariate analysis of variance of the five main categories of peer-related behaviors showed a reliable change with age, F (10, 46) = 2.06, $p < .05$. At all ages a prominent activity was watching the peer. Distant social responses were more frequent at each age than physical contact, but neither changed reliably with age. Vocalizing and smiling were the most frequent of the distant social responses; touching, the most frequent form of physical contact, especially at the youngest age. The behaviors related to the peer that changed with age were those that involved the play materials. The frequency of both contact with the same play material and direct involvement in the peer's play increased reliably, F (2, 27) = 4.77, $p < .02$; F (2, 27) = 8.42, $p < .001$, respectively.

Of the behaviors composing direct involvement in the peer's play, four showed orderly increases in frequency with age—imitation of the peer's activity, taking a toy from the peer, struggling over a toy, and coordinating activities with the toys. Five of the behaviors composing direct involvement in the peer's play—offering a toy, accepting a toy, taking a toy, taking over a toy, and struggling over a toy—concern the exchange or attempted exchange of play material between the two children. These exchange activities considered together occurred during an average of 1.9, 3.2, and 5.6 of the 40 intervals at the three

Table 16.1 Frequency of Peer-Related Activities

	M for each age group			
Behavior	10–12 months	16–18 months	22–24 months	F
Watch	18.3	19.2	15.9	<1
Distant social response	3.5	3.9	5.2	<1
Vocalize	1.7	1.5	3.1	
Smile	1.8	2.8	1.9	
Laugh	.0	.3	1.2	
Fuss	.0	.0	.1	
Cry	.0	.0	.0	
Gesture	.0	.1	.0	
Physical contact	2.0	.8	1.1	1.14
Touch	2.0	.5	.6	
Strike	.1	.3	.5	
Same play material	6.5	6.8	14.1	4.77*
Direct involvement in play	2.6	4.4	9.9	8.42**
Imitate	.9	1.3	2.0	
Show a toy	.2	.0	.3	
Offer a toy	.7	.8	.8	
Accept a toy	.3	.5	.2	
Take a toy	.1	.1	.6	
Take over a toy	.4	1.0	.8	
Struggle	.4	.8	3.2	
Coordinate	.0	.0	2.5	

* $p < .02$
** $p < .001$

ages and thus accounted for the greatest proportion of the activities composing direct involvement in play. Imitation by the focus child was the next most frequent activity across the ages, followed by coordinated play. Note, however, that imitation was recorded only when the focus child imitated the peer and not when the peer imitated him; the best estimate, then, of the frequency of imitation by either child is twice the frequencies tabulated, or 1.8, 2.6, and 4.0 periods at the increasing ages. Taking a toy and strugling—negative social responses according to Maudry and Nekula (1939)—together accounted for far less than half of the direct involvement in the peer's play at all ages.

Most of the peer-related behaviors were divided for purposes of comparison into Maudry and Nekula's (1939) positive and negative social reactions. Smile, laugh, vocalize, gesture, touch, show a toy, imitate, offer a toy, accept a toy, and coordinate toy activities comprise the positive reactions.

Fuss, cry, strike, take a toy, take over a toy, and struggle comprise the negative reactions.

At all ages positive responses far outweighed negative ones, and both positive and negative responses increased with age.

Growth of Social Play

Figure 16.2 contrasts the subjects' social play with solitary play. Social play includes the prior categories of same play material and direct involvement in play with the peer, as well as play with the mothers. A multivariate analysis of variance of solitary play and social play showed a reliable change in behavior with age, F (4, 52) = 3.78, $p < .01$. Solitary play occurred in slightly more than a third of the periods at all ages; social play, in contrast, increased reliably with age, F (2, 27) = 5.42, $p < .01$, until by 2 years it occurred in 60 percent of the periods. The increase in social play resulted from the reliable increase in play with the peer (see figure 16.2B), F (2, 27) = 10.86, $p < .001$. Play with the mother reached a peak at 16 to 18 months, F (2, 27) = 3.28, $p = .05$; play with the new adult, that is, the other mother, was rare. By 2 years of age, then, most of the children's activities with toys also involved a person, and in this novel play setting, that person was more often the peer than the mother.

Discussion

The results showed that during the second year of life, children in a novel play seting turned less to their mothers and more and more to inanimate objects and their peers. Further, the children increasingly integrated their activities with toys and peers until, by 2 years of age, social play predominated. They touched the same objects as their peers, imitated their actions, exchanged toys, and coordinated their play to perform a common task or elaborate a social game.

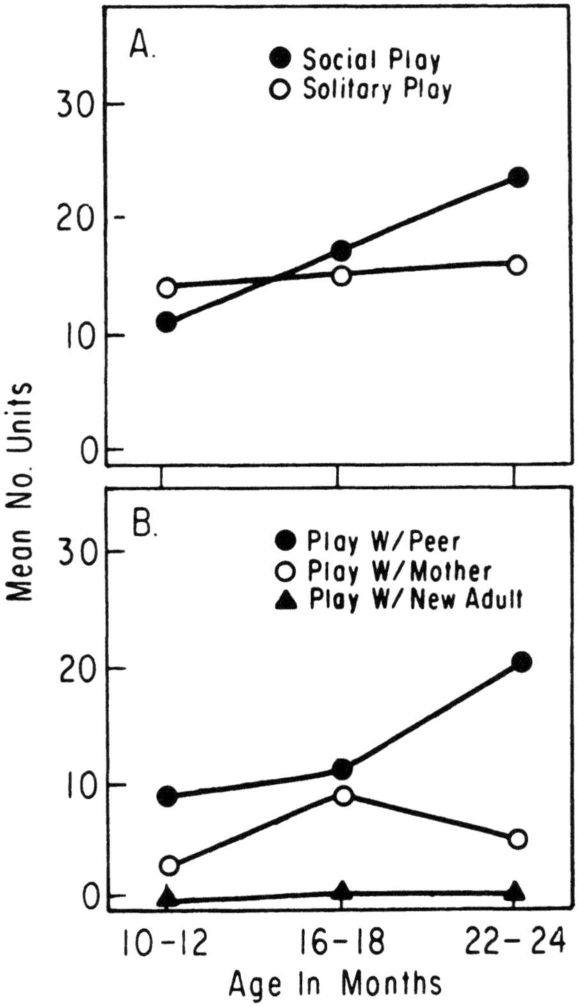

Figure 16.2. The Development of Social Play.

The current study leads to conclusions about the developmental course of peer interactions quite different from those of Maudry and Nekula (1939). At 10 to 12 months, ages at which Maudry and Nekula characterize infants as treating each other as an obstacle to play material, the children of the present study smiled and vocalized to each other, offered and accepted toys, and imitated each other; only infrequently did they struggle over toys or fuss. Further, rather than episodic, qualitative changes in reactions to peers, the present results suggest an orderly increase in the variety and frequency of social interactions between children—both the so-called negative and positive interactions. Of the numerous differences in methodology that might account for the contrasting pictures of social development, the most salient difference appears to be Maudry and Nekula's prompting of the children into interaction and the accompanying restriction of toy materials and alternative activities.

The integration of activities with toys and people during the second year of life highlights a central aspect of development. The responses we call social do not develop in a context devoid of inanimate objects; similarly those responses toward inanimate objects that we label exploration or play occur often in a social context. The mother, or attachment object, provides the setting for the infant's exploration of his inanimate world (e.g., Ainsworth & Wittig 1969; Rheingold 1969). Social objects, adults or children, also alter the stimulation that toys offer; they put toys in motion, make them do new things, and place them with other objects in new combinations. A toy on the ground does not equal a toy in the hand of a peer. On the other hand, nonsocial objects are vehicles for many forms of social interaction—for giving and taking, imitating, cooperating, or instructing. Smiling and vocalizing to persons or contacting them may be prominent early social behaviors, but other forms of social interaction require the child's integration of activities with things and people.

The children of all ages behaved toward one another not as children do with inanimate objects, but rather more as they do with familiar adults. The physical contact and manipulation characteristic of early activity with toys were minimal with the peer; rather the smiles, vocalizations, and offers of toys to the peer corresponded to behaviors seen with mothers (e.g., Rheingold 1973). A comparison, however, between play with the mother and direct play with the peer (the most nearly comparable categories of play) yields suggestive differences in the developmental course of these activities. At 10 to 12 months both were infrequent; by 16 to 18 months both were more frequent, but play with the mother exceeded that with the peer; and by 22 to

24 months play with the mother had declined in frequency, while direct play with the peer incrased markedly. Both the correspondence in forms of behavior toward the mother and the peer and the initial greater frequency of these behaviors toward the mother suggest that young children generalize to peers responses developed through interaction with familiar adults.

By 2 years of age, however, the children of the present study interacted more with the peer than with their mothers. The restrictive instructions to the mother and the short duration of the play period may have contributed to this preference, but the fact remains that with increasing age primate young turn progressively more to their peers in play (e.g., Harlow 1969; Heathers 1955). The question of what peers offer in contrast to familiar adults is an important one for the fuller understanding of early social behavior. Peers and adults seem to differ in their persistence and affective involvement in children's play and the contrast shifts during the child's development. Mothers and fathers initially invest great persistence, affect, and imagination in attempts to engage their young infants in play, but later in development peers often seem more ready than parents to follow through on a child's playful overtures. Still, peers have two other characteristics that warrant study: Their actions and reactions may be more novel than those of parents, and the activities of peers may be more easily duplicated than those of adults, who only with difficulty can behave as children do.

The present study, then, has demonstrated that home-reared children during the second year of life freely engage in a variety of social interactions with unfamiliar peers, interactions that resemble those with familiar adults more than those with inanimate objects. They smile, laugh, vocalize and gesture to one another, show and offer toys, imitate each other, struggle, and engage in reciprocal play. Thus, interactions with peers and with familiar adults appear closely intertwined in development. Yet as more and more of the children's play involved people, the social partner was more often the peer than the mother. This choice of the peer makes still more tenable the speculation that peers—even infant peers—make their own contribution to early human sociability.

17

Self, Other, and Fear

The Reaction of Infants to People

MICHAEL LEWIS AND
JEANNE BROOKS-GUNN

The fears that infants exhibit, as they relate to affective, cognitive, and social development, are important to study. Many have suggested that a fear of strangers may be an index of attachment. Although attachment has been defined as a positive approach to the mother as measured by proximal and distal behaviors during play (Coates, Anderson, & Hartup 1972; Lewis & Ban 1971) and reunion (Ainsworth et al. 1978; Goldberg & Lewis 1969; Schaffer & Emerson 1964), attachment may also be explored by examining the infant's responses to other persons, either when the mother is or is not present. Responses to strangers also allow us to study the child's social behavior and the categories into which young infants divide their social world (Brooks-Gunn & Lewis 1976; Lewis & Brooks-Gunn 1975).

Fear of the stranger may also be related to cognitive development. Indeed, Hebb (1946, 1949), Piaget (1952), and others (Schaffer, 1966) have argued that the relationship between fear and novelty is such that great amounts of discrepancy or novelty may result in a fear response when the organism is unable to assimilate a highly discrepant event. Moreover, increased cognitive capacity in all probability leads to greater differentiation among categories of persons.

Fear of strangers or stranger anxiety traditionally has been studied as an ethological phenomenon (Ainsworth & Bell 1970; Schaffer & Emerson 1964). This literature suggests that fear of strangers usually appears in the second half of the first year and extends long into the second year for some (Lewis & Rosenblum 1974). As an ethological-imprinting process, fear of strangers is a way of binding the infant to his caregiver. However, not all infants exhibit fear of strangers, as Rheingold and Eckerman (1971) first pointed out. Some infants (and perhaps the majority) show signs of wariness or differential smiling towards unfamiliar people, but not outright fear (Haviland & Lewis 1976; Lewis & Rosenblum 1974).

For all the current research on fear in infancy, there has been relatively little effort directed toward the social dimensions which elicit fear. While age of onset, number of infants exhibiting fear, and specific fears of animate objects have received the most attention, we are interested in the infant's response to different categories of people. Morgan and Ricciutti (1969) studied infants' responses to male and female strangers and found that infants were more negative in the presence of males. Although we do not know about the other characteristics of the strangers (height, shape, presence of facial hair, hair length) in their study, it seems that differential responses were a function of the nature of the social event, in this case, a gender difference. It is to this finding and to an observation of an 8-month-old female that our study is directed. We observed that an approach by an adult stranger produced extreme fear in the infant. She screamed, cried, and tried desperately to escape. But when a stranger 3- or 4-years-old approached her, she smiled, cooed, and reached. Why should this be when both persons were equally strange to her? Would children who were generally fearful respond similarly? What does this mean for the cognitive functioning of the infant, let alone its significance for any theory of social relations? As a first step, this casual observation had to be repeated and extended.

Method

Subjects and Procedure

In the present study we were interested in the infants' responses to five different social events: a strange adult male and female of the same physical size, a strange female child 4 years of age, the infant's mother, and a mirror representation of the infant subject. Twenty-four infants ranging from 7 to 19 months of age were placed one at a time in a pleasant, carpeted, furnished room. Only infants who were first-born or who had siblings over 5 years of age were included; 20 were first-born and 4 had siblings over 5.

All infants were Caucasian, were healthy, and came from lower middle to upper middle-class families. The infant was seated in an infant tenda facing a door about 15 feet away. The mother sat next to the child. The first of three strangers knocked on the door. The mother said "come in," and the stranger entered at the far end of the room and slowly walked toward the infant. Having reached the infant, the stranger touched the infant's hand. Throughout the episode, the stranger smiled but did not vocalize (since we could not "train" our child stranger to vocalize in a set fashion). Movements were deliberately slow to avoid eliciting startle responses. After touching the infant, the stranger slowly turned, walked to the door, and left the room. The entire sequence took approximately 15 seconds. The second and third strangers followed the same procedure. There was approximately a 2-minute wait between visits or until the infant was quiet.

The order of appearance of the strangers was counterbalanced across subjects and no order or order x stranger effects were found. After the stranger approached, the mother went to the door and walked toward and away from the infant just as the strangers had. For the self condition, the infants saw themselves in a mirror. Rather than having the novelty of the mirror approaching the infant, the infant approached the mirror. To do this, the mother moved the tenda so that it was directly in front of a mirror placed at the opposite end of the room. She slowly moved the tenda toward the mirror so that the infant was able to see his or her reflection without observing the mother. When the tenda touched the mirror, the mother moved away. The order was counterbalanced for the mother and self conditions; again, no order effects were found.

Measures

Three behavioral scales—facial expression, vocalization, and motor activity—were used to rate the infants' reactions to the stranger conditions. Distance 1, the farthest distance, was when the stranger entered; distance 2 (middle) was when the social event was in the middle of the room; distance 3 (close) was when the event was 3 feet from the infant; and distance 4 (touch) was when the event touched the infant. Since there was almost no vocalizing, crying, or fretting, the data from the vocalization scale will not be presented.

Results

Social Condition and Distance Effects

The mean data for the facial and motor scales by distance, stranger condition, and age of infant will be presented. For all of the figures, a score of 3 indicates a neutral response; 1 a negative response (puckering frown, turning from the stranger and toward the mother); and 5 a positive response (broad smile, reaching toward the social event). Figure 17.1 presents the mean of the two scales by distance and social condition.

As can be seen, affective social differentiation increased with proximity. No affect differences toward the various social events were found when the person was at the farthest end of the room, while differences appeared as the person approached. The persons differed in their effect on the infant's positive and negative affect. The male and female adult strangers elicited the most (and only) negative responses; the child stranger elicited a some-

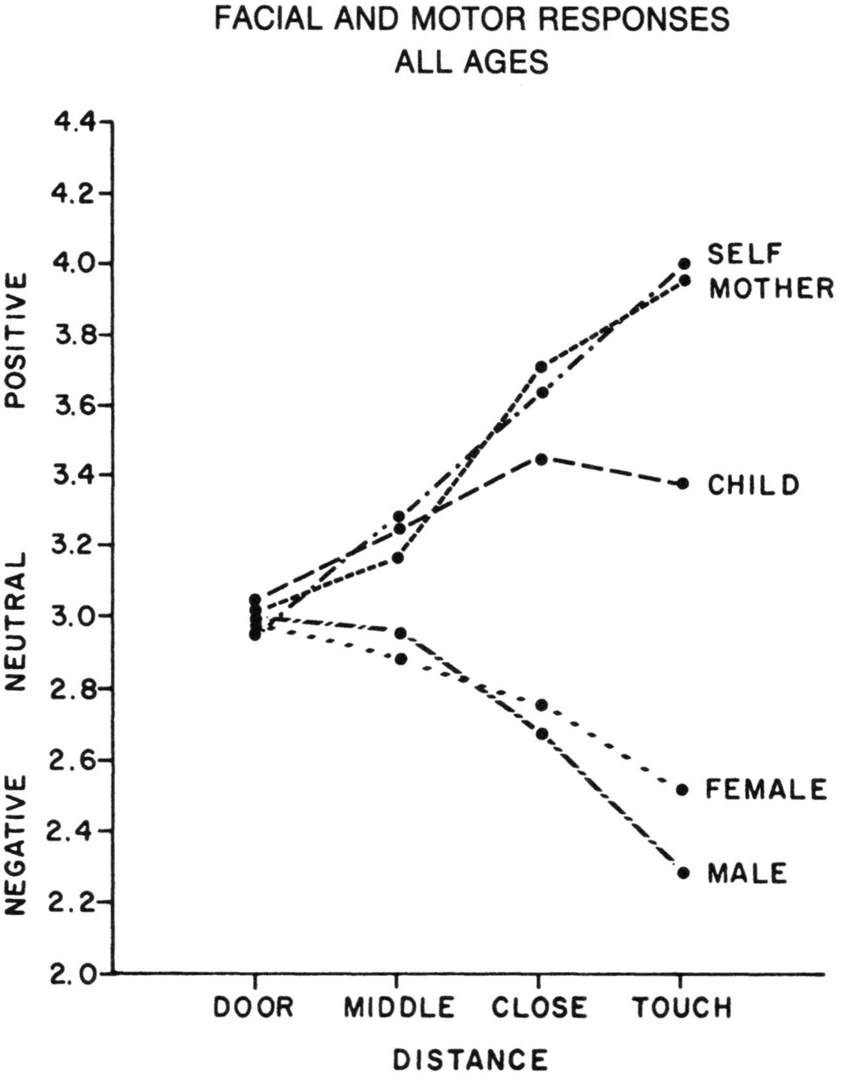

Figure 17.1. Mean facial and motor responses to the five social events for all infants. A score of 3 indicates a neutral response. Scores less than and more than 3 indicate negative and positive response respectively.

what positive response; and the mother and self elicited the most positive responses. In a two-way analysis of variance (social conditions and distance), the social condition, distance, and stimulus x distance interaction effects all were significant ($F = 11.25, p < .001$; $F = 16.10, p < .001$; $F = 18.04, p < .001$, respectively).

These findings are consistent with Morgan and Ricciutti's (1969) findings that infants do not exhibit either positive or negative responses when a person is far away but do so as the person approaches or is a close proximity. These responses are a compromise between the need to flee (something strange can hurt) and the need to experience newness in order to alter cognitive structures. The child's strategy might be to *stay and attend as long as the event does not get close; if it approaches, withdraw*. Fear and negative affect may be in the service of this escape behavior.

Subject Age Effects

Differentiation of responses to the various social events was also related to subject age as well as to distance. When the sample was divided by median age, 12 subjects were between 7 and 11.5 months of age and 12 infants were between 12 and 19 months of age. We realize that the small sample size and the arbitrary division of the infants into two age groups limits generalization; however, interesting age differences emerged. While the patterns for the two age levels were similar, older infants exhibited a greater range of responses than did the younger ones. The older infants were more positive to the self, the mother, and the child stranger and more negative toward the female and male adult strangers. Statistically, infants over and under 1 year of age responded significantly differently to the adults (t test, $p < .05$) and only somewhat differently to the mother and self (t test, $p < .10$). These age differences were not found for the total approach scores but only for the distances 3 and 4 approach scores sums (when the social event was in close proximity). The greater experience and presumably greater cognitive sophistication of the older infants did not result in more prompt affective responses. In brief, approach determines the timing while age affects the intensity of the response (especially negative responses).

Subject Gender Effects

The sex of the infant was not related to the affective response to social events, with the exception of responses to the adult male stranger. While the infants in general were more negative in the presence of the male stranger, this effect was only seen in the female infants.

Discussion

Strangeness as a Predictor of Negative Affect

How are we to account for the negative affect directed toward the adult strangers and the positive affect directed toward the child stranger and to the mother and self? Since we would expect fear of strangers, the negative expression toward the adult strangers comes as no surprise. However, if it is strangeness alone that elicits fear or negative affect, why do we see no fear (and in fact, see positive responding) toward the child stranger? This brings into question the whole incongruity hypothesis. The incongruity argument as it relates to affect states that events that are highly incongruous will produce little fear. For example, the head of a monkey (apart from the body) shown to other monkeys produces extreme fear, presumably because of its incongruity (Hebb 1946). If the judgment of congruity is made with the mother as the referent, then the strange female is least incongruent, the strange male more so, and the strange female child most. Thus, the child stranger should produce the most fear. In fact, the child stranger produces no fear but, in fact, produces a positive affect. Therefore, we suggest that incongruity may not be the sole determinant of fear. On the other hand, the mother may not be the only referent for infants. Remember that infants also show positive affect to themselves. We will return to this issue shortly.

These data also suggest that we reconsider our formulation about infants' fear of strangers. It now becomes clear that not all strange social events that approach infants will elicit the same degree of negative affect. That is, strangeness per se is not a sufficient elicitor of fear or wariness, and multidimensional determinants are necessary; strangeness is necessary but not sufficient. What are the characteristics of the child stranger that *do not* elicit fearful responses? Two appear most likely; the first is size. Clearly, the child stranger is smaller than the adults; also, the child stranger is closer in size to the infant, especially one sitting in a baby tenda. Ethologically, it makes sense to postulate that an organism should be more frightened of strange things that are bigger than itself than of those that are the same size or smaller than itself. Same size or smaller things are less likely or able to hurt. The second dimension is the differential facial configuration between a young child and an adult; Lorenz (1943) has postulated that adults are very responsive to babyishness, preferring pictures and figure drawings of young animals and humans who have round features. Perhaps this is the cue. When a 12-month-old looks through magazines and newspapers containing pictures of adults (pictures that are, of course, not life size) it has been observed that he will say the widely used word "baby" as he points to the figures, suggesting that he is responding to the size of the picture rather than the facial configuration. Whatever the explanation of why the infants were not upset by the child stranger, it is clear that a simple incongruity explanation fails to satisfy the data and that the space of social strangeness is multidimensional, unfamiliarity being just one dimension.

The Concept of Self

The infant's highly positive response to the mother was as we expected; however, the equally positive response to self in the mirror was somewhat more interesting. By using the term "self," we have been making an explicit assumption, one which was quite intentional. There is relatively little information on infants' responses to mirrors, but the anecdotal evidence that does exist indicates that even at ages earlier than those of the children in the experiment, there is an intense positive affective response to the mirror. In a study of 4-month-olds by Rheingold (1971), further evidence for the positive effect of seeing oneself in the mirror was reported. These infants showed more smiling to a mirror image than to motion pictures or slides of an infant or to nonsocial stimuli.

Can one talk about the concept of the self at such early ages? Consider two aspects of the self: the first and most common is the categorical self (I am female, or I am intelligent, or I am big or small, or I am capable); the second and by far the more primitive, is the existential statement "I am." The basic notion of self—probably as differentiated from other (either as object or person, the mother being the most likely other person)—must develop first. There is no reason not to assume that it develops from birth and that even in the early months some notion of self exists. We would argue that this nonevaluative, existential self is developed from the consistency and regularity of, and feedback resultant from, the infant's actions and their outcome in the world. Self is differentiated by reafferent (or information) feedback; for example, each time a certain set of muscles operate (eyes close), it becomes black (cannot see). That is, the immediacy, simultaneity, and regularity of action and outcome produces differentiation and self. The action of touching the hot stove and the immediacy of the pain tells me it's my hand that is on the stove. This self is further reinforced if, when I remove my hand, the pain ceases. Infants' worlds are full of such relationships, and they vary from the infants' own action on objects to their relationships with caregivers and others. In social interactions, the highly directed energy of the caregiver (touch, smile, look, etc.) is contingent and specific to infant action (smile, coo, etc.).

Fear and the Concept of Self

Is our understanding of the phenomenon of fear helped by evoking the concept of self? We would argue yes. The notion of self seems relevant with respect to our findings. Perhaps female infants are more frightened than male infants of male adult strangers because the male infant recognizes that the male adult is more like himself. The specific category of self in this case may be gender. The Money, Hampson, and Hampson (1957) data on sexual identity and gender anomalies suggest that infants under 18 months of life may already possess this category, becoming disturbed if sex reassignments are made after the first year of life.

That there was a positive response to the child stranger and negative responses to the adult strangers is difficult to explain in any incongruity hypothesis unless we consider that the referent for the social comparison does not always have to be the infant's mother. There could be multiple referents, one of them being the mother, another being the self. Perhaps the positive response to the child stranger was produced because the infants used themselves as referents and, finding the child to be like themselves, were therefore not afraid. In this case the categorical dimension of self may have to do with size. "I am small vis-à-vis other social events and the child is also small and, therefore, like me."

In this discussion of fear, two major theoretical positions have been evoked and it would help to clarify matters by stating them explicitly. These are the ethological and cognitive approaches. The ethological position rests less (if at all) on a cognitive approach and more on an imprinting or innate releasing mechanism approach. The argument for the present data would be as follows: the infant is imprinted on parents and all others are perceived as strange. When the strange event is at a distance, "observe closely, but do not flee." When the strange event approaches, "flee." The only caveat would be that strange has to be bigger than the organism. This model requires the use of no or little cognitive process, and following the ethological approach, is rather mechanistic in nature.

The cognitive approach, on the other hand, invokes concepts such as incongruity, novelty and familiarity, and schema. These all rest on the interaction between the organism's past and present experiences. Moreover, the cognitive approach requires the introduction of such processes as object permanence, at least in terms of remembering the mother. This approach stresses that the child's response to strangers is a part of the larger emerging cognitive functions. We would extend this position by considering the concept of self and using it as an additional referent in terms of social interactions and cognitions. While the ethological approach has intrinsic appeal—especially since it evokes a biological simplicity—it is difficult for us to consider infants not responding through the use of the elaborate cognitive functions which we know are already available to them.

PART V

Postnatal Influences

Within and Beyond the Family

Having considered the course of cognitive and socioemotional development during infancy in the two preceding sections, we present here articles on the topic of early experience. These seven articles focus upon familial and extrafamilial influences on infant development. In the first essay, Leon Yarrow and his colleagues empirically examine relationships between early home environment and cognitive/motivational development. Detailed observations of mother-infant interaction, along with developmental assessments of infant functioning, reveal that caregivers who are positively oriented toward their infants, and responsive to them when they are five months of age, have infants who at six months look especially competent. More important than the documentation of these relationships, though, are the explanations of psychological processes that Yarrow et al. offer to account for these and other findings. It is these analyses that the attentive reader will be especially interested in.

The second article is concerned with early maternal influences on social development. Working from a perspective that emphasizes the harmony rather than the conflict that can exist in the socialization process, Stayton, Hogan, and Ainsworth present data to support their hypothesis that infant obedience and cooperation is a natural outgrowth of a sensitive caregiving experience. These findings, as the authors themselves stress, pose a serious challenge to developmental theories that construe socialization as a struggle in which the young child's yearnings are in conflict with those of the social world in which s/he must learn to live. The fact that cognitive as well as social development outcomes are found in the study to be related to sensitive mothering underscores again a point made throughout this volume—that cognitive and social development are inextricably intertwined in the human infant.

While the early mother-infant relationship has been long recognized for its developmental importance, it is only in recent years that systematic attention has been paid to the early father-child relationship. Evidence of this interest is documented in the third article, in which Allison Clarke-Stewart examines not only the similarities and differences in the mother-infant and father-infant relationships but also the differential and combined influence of the two parents on infant cognitive and social development. Clarke-Stewart also presents evidence highlighting the influence of the father on the mother-child relationship, an influence which is considered especially important because it underscores the fact that the child develops in a family system. Thus, what transpires between mother and child can be affected by what transpires elsewhere in the family.

Consideration of the family system's perspective, which emphasizes the interdependence of relationships within the family, draws attention to the need to study the marital relationship in order to understand the infant's early experiences and how they affect his subsequent development. For the most part, psychologists have failed in this regard. Indeed, with the exception of studies of divorce, developmentalists have failed to adopt a truely family perspective in their investigations of infancy.

In the case of one researcher, however, this is notably untrue. At an international conference in 1975, Frank Pedersen presented a paper, published for the first time in this volume, that can only be considered as ahead of its time. Not only does Pedersen discuss in this article the indirect role that fathers may play in influencing infant functioning by affecting maternal attitudes and behavior, but he presents data suggesting that the quality of the marital relationship may influence the sensitivity and skill with which mothers care for their babies. While this study is by no means definitive, it is important in showing how consideration of a family system's perspective, and especially mothers' and fathers' relations with each other as husband and wife, may support or undermine the care, known to be developmentally influential, that the infant receives.

Next, Michael Lamb presents a study of 18-month-old infants and their preschool siblings. His data and approach clearly mesh with a family system's perspective in recognizing that the child's world is made up of people, and that his development is influenced by persons other than his two parents. Most intriguing in this study is Lamb's finding that preschool siblings serve as role models for their younger brothers and sisters, who regularly imitate their activities. Also important is Lamb's suggestion that preschoolers offer their younger siblings something distinct from what their mothers and fathers do.

Thus, the first five articles amply document the importance of experience *in* the family for the young infant. The remaining two readings highlight the significance of events occurring *beyond* the family. Specifically, they deal with two contemporary issues that undoubtedly exert an impact not only upon familial processes but also on infant development—maternal employment and day care. In this day and age when ever-increasing numbers of women are entering the labor force when their children are quite young, and when many of these children are being placed in supplementary child care arrangements, the effects of maternal employment and day care are becoming extremely important concerns.

In her paper dealing with maternal employment, Sarale Cohen reports a study that compares patterns of mother-child interaction among toddlers whose mothers were working or were remaining at home to rear them. Results revealed several differences that appear to favor those children whose mothers were not employed, and support for this interpretation is provided by data on developmental assessments that enabled Cohen to compare the cognitive functioning of the two groups of infants.

These findings, however, should not be considered definitive with regard to the issue of the effect of maternal employment, as they derive from only a single investigation of one small sample of children. Whether or not results such as these can be replicated will determine, in part, the conclusions that are eventually reached on this important issue. Furthermore, there can be little doubt that the effects of a mother's working are mediated by a host of other factors, including her attitude toward working. And, in this regard, some evidence does exist which demonstrates that, at least with older children, when mothers do what they desire to do (be it stay home or work), their children develop best. Thus, it may not be employment or nonemployment that is the critical factor in determining the influence of the mother's working on infant development.

Another factor that must be considered in addition to mothers' attitudes toward work is the kind and quality of care infants are provided when their mothers are away. In this section's final article, Belsky and Steinberg's critical and authoritative review of the effects of day care is reprinted. In it they summarize data on the effects of supplementary child care on cognitive, emotional, and social development. While they essentially give day care a clean bill of health regarding its effects on development in infancy and the early childhood years, they make two important qualifying comments. First, they note that little evidence exists on the long-term effects of out-of-home care; and second, they observe that most day care studied to date has been of very high quality. Their generalizations, then, are applicable only to other high-quality rearing environments.

18

Dimensions of Early Stimulation and Their Differential Effects on Infant Development

LEON J. YARROW, JUDITH L. RUBENSTEIN
FRANK A. PEDERSEN, AND
JOSEPH J. JANKOWSKI

To some extent, experimental studies have confirmed the general premise that marked trauma and extreme deprivation can have significant effects. The impact of less extreme variations in experiences, experiences within the "normal" range, is much less clear. This is due in part to a lack of differentiation of environments, and to our difficulties in describing and measuring with any degree of precision the dimensions of natural environments. In this study we have looked at a range of variation in experiences of five- to six-month-old infants on a concrete behavioral level, and have conceptualized these discrete behaviors.

Our major objectives in this study were: (1) to differentiate the natural environment in conceptually meaningful terms through detailed analysis of the caretaker's behavior and properties of the proximal inanimate stimuli in the infant's environment; and (2) to determine the extent to which separate dimensions or components of these variables (e.g., variety, complexity, and responsiveness of inanimate stimuli; level and variety of social stimulation; and the expression of positive affect) have different orders of relationships to the development of early infant functions.

This study represents a convergence of applied and theoretical interests. We were especially interested in assessing the impact on development of so-called "disadvantaged" environments in early infancy. Limited observational data are available on mother-infant interaction in disadvantaged groups. Moreover, we thought environmental effects might be highlighted in these settings. Our sample, however, represents a wide continuum on environmental variables. Therefore, the implications of this research go beyond disadvantaged or depriving environments; the findings have relevance for understanding a broad range of environmental influences on development.

Method

The sample consisted of 41 black infants, 21 boys and 20 girls, who had been cared for by a stable "primary caretaker." The mother was the primary caretaker in 30 cases, a relative (usually the maternal grandmother) in 6 cases, and an unrelated babysitter in 5 cases. Of this group, 34 were recruited through two public well-baby clinics. Their fathers had completed from 6 to 12 years of school, with a mean of 10.9 years, and were engaged in primarily semi-skilled and unskilled occupations. To extend the range on the environmental variables, 7 black infants were obtained through a private group medical program. These families were all intact, and the fathers' education ranged from one year of college through graduate school; the mean educational level was 14.6 years. All infants were of normal birth weight, were free from gross complications in pregnancy or delivery, and were screened by a pediatrician to eliminate cases in which there were any indications of neurological damage.

The basic data were obtained through time-sampling observations in the home when the infants were 5 months of age. The mother or baby's caretaker was encouraged to go about her usual activities. Two home observations about a week apart were conducted; each involved 3 hours of time-sampling while the baby was awake. The time-sampling cycle consisted of a 30-second observation period and a 60-second recording period repeated through 120 cycles each day. There are a total of 240 time-sample units, or 6 hours, for each child and caretaker.

Approximately 60 categories of events were monitored in each interval. Selected infant behaviors observed included positive vocalizations, fussing or irritable vocalizations, and whether the infant was engaging in focused manipulation of play objects or directing his visual attention to the mother. Approximately 45 categories of caretaker behavior were recorded describing aspects of social stimulation. There were, in addition, several time-sample measures of the proximal inanimate environment. The categories of social stimulation can be classified in the following areas: (1) *Sensory modality* of social stimulation (e.g., visual, auditory, tactile, and kinesthetic stimulation, as exemplified by looking at, talking to, and holding the baby); (2) The *intensity* or rate of stimulus change (for example, passive holding is distinguished from active touching or moving the baby); (3) Whether stimulation is *contingent* on certain infant behaviors (for example, social soothing in response to distress states, contingent vocal response to the infant's positive vocalizations); and (4) The *type* or class of behavior the caretaker is attemptimg to evoke (for example, the attainment of motor skills such as postural control or locomotion, or fostering interest in play materials by highlighting the properties of toys or positioning them for the baby). In addition, ratings were made of the caretaker's expression of positive affect toward the infant and contingency of response to distress.

Environmental variables. Our basic strategy in choosing variables for differentiated analysis of the natural environment was to order the infant's experiences in terms of a conceptual framework. Level of social stimulation was a composite of the amount and intensity of stimulation by the caretaker. We obtained through time sampling the frequency with which the mother was within view of and within reach of the infant, and the frequency with which she talked to the infant, touched or held him, or engaged him in vigorous play. These discrete behaviors were weighted on a five-point scale so that vigorous play involving intense stimulation and several modalities received a higher score than stimulation of low intensity in one modality, such as touching the baby.

Variety of social stimulation is an unweighted sum of different types of social stimulation. Examples of these are play, encouraging motor responses, presentation of play objects, the range of affect which the caretaker exhibited, and the number of different physical settings in which social stimulation occurred.

Two indices of contingency were used: (1) frequency of contingent responses to positive vocalizations by the infant obtained through time-sampling (interobserver reliability .96); and (2) contingency of response to distress, a 5-point rating scale based on latency of response to the infant's distress signals. These variables are derived from operant learning theory (Gewirtz 1969) and other formulations (Ainsworth 1967; Lewis & Goldberg 1969) emphasizing the importance of early intervention in distress states.

The variable, expression of positive affect, was based on ratings by the observers following the time-sampling observations. It is a measure of characteristic level of demonstrativeness of the mother or caretaker.

The Infant Variables

The dependent variables were derived from two procedures: a research form, the Bayley Scales of Infant Development (administered in the fifth month), and a structured situational test measuring exploratory behavior and preference for novel stimuli (administered in the sixth month). In addition to the Mental Developmental Index and Psychomotor Developmental Index which the Bayley yields, eight more differentiated clusters were developed. Items were grouped on the basis of their apparent conceptual coherence. Split-half and part-whole analyses provided a statistical basis for further refinement. The final split-half reliabilities ranged from .74 to .92. The clusters include: *Social Responsiveness, Language, Fine Motor, Gross Motor*, and four measures that we considered indices of cognitive-motivational functions—*Goal Orientation, Reaching* and *Grasping, Secondary Circular Reaction,* and *Object Permanence.* Another cluster, *Problem Solving*—a measure of rudimentary means-ends relationships—was developed from four supplementary items administered after the Bayley Test.

The procedure for measuring exploratory behavior and preference for novel stimuli, functions that we also labeled cognitive-motivational, involves presenting the baby with an attractive, novel toy—a bell—for 10 minutes. The amount of exploratory interest shown by looking and manipulating was recorded. Then a series of 10 new toys were presented one at a time for 1-minute intervals together with the bell, which had become more familiar. Preference for novel stimuli was expressed by measures of differential looking or manipulation, that is, the difference between time directed to the novel toy vs. the more familiar bell.

Results

Differentiation of the environment. Table 18.1 indicates the interrelationships among the social variables. Level, variety, and positive affect are all rather strongly interrelated. In fact, level has considerable generality with all other social stimulation var-

Table 18.1 Interrelationships Among the Social Variables

	Social			
	Variety	Positive Affect	Cont. R. to Pos. Voc.	Cont. R. to Distress
Social				
Level	.76	.62	.64	.53
Variety		.64	.45	.48
Positive Affect			.51	.23
Contingent Response to Positive Vocalization				.31
Contingent Response to Distress				

for p = .05, one-tailed test, r = .26.

iables. In regard to the two contingency measures, there is a relatively low relationship between the frequency measure, contingent response to positive vocalization and the latency measure, contingent response to distress ($r = .31$). This suggests that maternal responsiveness is itself not a highly general trait.

Relations Between the Social Environment and Infant Functioning. Both level and variety of social stimulation are thought of as having an arousal function, serving to activate the infant and increase his responsiveness to the environment. The general pattern of relationships seen in table 18.2 is quite similar for

Table 18.2 Correlations Between Social Stimulation Variables and Infant Functioning

	Social Stimulation Variables				
Infant Functioning	Level	Variety	Positive Affect	Cont. R. Pos. Voc.	Cont. R. Distress
General Status					
Mental Developmental Index	.32**	.34*	.23	—	.32*
Psychomotor Developmental Index	—	.23	—	—	.37*
Social Responsiveness	.35*	.34*	.26*	.22	—
Language					
Vocalize to Bell	—	.31*	.24	.30*	—
Language Quality	—	—	—	—	—
Motor Development					
Gross	—	—	—	—	.28*
Fine	—	.26*	—	—	.33*
Goal-Director Behaviors					
Goal Orientation	.45**	.48**	.30*	—	.38**
Reaching	.25	.28	—	—	.29*
Secondary Circular Reaction	.32*	.35*	.30*	—	.30*
Cognitive Functions					
Problem Solving	.21	.20	—	—	—
Object Permanence	.31*	.47**	—	—	—
Exploratory Behavior					
Looking at Bell	—	—	—	−.37	—
Manipulating Bell	—	.32	—	—	.21
Looking at Novel	—	—	—	—	—
Manipulating Novel	—	—	.28*	.31*	.24

* $p < .05$; one-tailed test
** $p < .01$; one-tailed test
– indicates r less than .20.

these two variables, although a greater number of significant correlations are found with variety.

The variables were defined quite differently. Level is defined in terms of characteristics of the stimuli themselves, amount weighted by different degrees of intensity. Variety was defined in terms of the types of behavior elicited by the caretaker and the different physical settings where interaction occurred. It is the frequency of interactive play, motor training, presentation and highlighting of play objects, and the number of changes in the location of interaction with the baby, such as an infant seat, the caretaker's lap, or the floor. The essence of variety is the encouragement of more differentiated responses on the part of the infant, whereas level is defined in terms of the stimulus characteristics.

As with level and variety, contingent response to distress is also significantly related to the Mental Developmental Index and to the measures of goal-directed behavior. These results seem to support the Ainsworth (1967) or the Lewis and Goldberg (1969) interpretation of what happens when one responds to the infant's cry; relatively early intervention in distress states may have a general facilitating effect, either by freeing the infant to respond to external stimuli or by making him aware of a contingent relationship with the caretaker.

There are two language measures. Vocalize to Bell is a measure of *amount* of vocalization obtained during the test of exploratory behavior, the 10-minute period when the infant had the interesting toy. Its significant relationship with the mother's contingent response to infant vocalization has special conceptual interest. This relationship found in the natural environment adds to the generalizability to life settings of the operant laboratory studies of the social reinforcement of vocalization rates (Rheingold, Gewirtz, & Ross 1959; Weisberg 1963; Todd & Palmer 1968). Another measure, the mother's spontaneous vocalizations (that is, total vocalization minus contingent vocalization) was not related to the infant's vocal output. This finding, as well as the lack of relationship to the other measure of contingency, underscores the specificity of this effect and buttresses the operant learning interpretation.

The second language measure is a cluster of 8 Bayley items dealing with the qualitative aspects of language. The measure was not related to any environmental variables. Although language quality at 5 to 6 months may be more important conceptually than amount of vocalization, it is probably too unstable developmentally or too complex to measure adequately with a few text items.

More evidence of differential effects is seen in relation to Social Responsiveness. This cluster of 8 Bayley items includes vocalizing to a social stimulus, anticipatory adjustment to lifting, enjoying frolic play, and approaching and smiling to a mirror image. Instigating stimuli, that is, level, variety, and expression of positive affect, are all significantly correlated with social responsiveness; whereas the soothing stimuli, contingent response to distress, are unrelated to social responsiveness.

The strongest grouping of significant relationships is in the cognitive-motivational set called Goal-Directed Behaviors. Goal Orientation is a cluster of 6 Bayley items, primarily motivational in nature, including such behaviors as persistent and purposeful attempts to secure objects just out of reach. This measure has very high generality with many other dependent variables; it correlates .86 with the total Bayley Mental Developmental Index, higher than any other cluster. The results suggest that motivational differences in infants are particularly sensitive to the social environment.

The cluster Reaching and Grasping consists of nine Bayley items and emphasizes especially visual-motor coordination and fine motor skills in transactions with play objects. it probably has more of a skill emphasis than other variables in this group, and that may account for the weaker relationships.

Secondary Circular Reaction, as defined by Piaget, is the repetition of behavior which produces interesting results. It reflects an intentionality to maintain interesting activities, and it is thought of as a precursor of instrumental behavior requiring an appreciation of means-ends relationships. The cluster consisted of only two items, banging in play and enjoying sound production. Despite the sharp restriction in range of the dependent variable, there are four correlations significant at the .05 level.

A supplementary test item with high face validity was also devised for measuring secondary circular reactions; the results were essentially the same as for the Bayley cluster.

Sex differences. Although results have been reported for the group as a whole, the data have also been analyzed separately for males and females. Generally, the direction of the relationships tends to be similar for boys and girls. However, the magnitude of relationships between environmental and infant variables is higher for females.

Discussion

Several issues important for developmental theory and research are highlighted by these findings. We have shown that the natural environment of the young infant can be differentiated into many discrete behaviors of the caretaker.

Another issue highlighted by the findings of this study concerns the level at which one characterizes environments. The findings underscore the inadequacy of global characterizations of environments, and emphasize the value of differentiating the dimensions and characteristics of stimulation.

A third issue has to do with the simple correlational model we have used. We recognize that looking at relationships between single variables is a very simple model that ignores the realities of environment-child interaction. Although there are many significant correlations between environmental variables and infant characteristics, the magnitude of many of the correlations is not very high. These associations exceed chance expectations and, in general, are consistent with theoretical assumptions, but they do not permit predictions with any high degree of accuracy. It is likely that these environmental variables interact in many complex ways. We cannot conclude that any single variable alone is decisive for any particular infant function. It is meaningful, however, to ask to what extent a given environmental variable makes a special contribution to some aspect of infant functioning.

We also need to ask more complex questions, such as: whether certain environmental variables may be interchangeable; whether certain combinations of variables are additive in their effects; and to what extent certain variables interact to strengthen or diminish each other's impact. We must also recognize that the relationship between environmental variables and infant behavior is not a simple unidirectional one. There is a reciprocal interaction between infant characteristics and environmental events. It is likely that an active and responsive infant elicits more social response from others as well as greater inanimate stimulation than a lethargic, withdrawn infant.

We have been particularly interested in the group of infant behaviors that we have called cognitive-motivational functions. One striking finding of this study is the extent to which these functions seem to be amenable to environmental influences in early infancy. These results support Provence and Lipton's (1961) impressions that motivational functions may be more vulnerable to depriving institutional environments than are specific emerging skills.

Motivation, as we have used it, is not an abstract intervening variable. It refers to clearly specified behaviors, such as reaching persistently for objects, attempting to have an effect on and elicit responses from objects, showing preferential attention to the manipulating novel objects. These behaviors might be considered expressions of the infant's motivation to assimilate, to learn about, and to master the environment. They may be viewed as an early expression of a competence or an effectance motive (White 1959). The importance of these relationships lies in their convergence with a number of theoretical formulations based primarily on laboratory studies. Lewis and Goldberg (1969) have formulated a "generalized expectancy model," emphasizing the role of contingent mother-infant interaction in the development of the child's belief that he can affect his environment, that he can bring about reinforcement by his actions. Watson (1966) speaks of "contingency awareness" as a precondition for later learning. The common thread in these formulations is the active, information-processing organism, initiating transactions with the environment and in turn being influenced by these transactions.

One last point in regard to the significance of motivational functions. It is likely that the infant's orientation to objects and to people very early becomes part of a feedback system with the environment. His smiling, vocalizing, and reaching out to people and his visually attending to and manipulating objects tend to be self-reinforcing and thus, to some extent, self perpetuating. These behaviors become part of a system of reciprocal interactions which may characterize a given infant's transactions with the environment over a long period of time. This orientation to the world may be a more consistent and more significant characteristic of the young infant than any specific cognitive ability. We might speculate that the infant's orientation to his environments adds to the continuity of his experiences. If this is so, then the fact that these aspects of functioning seem to be related to identifiable aspects of the environment during the first six months may have great significance not only for developmental theory, but for intervention programs as well.

19

Infant Obedience and Maternal Behavior

The Origins of Socialization Reconsidered

DONELDA J. STAYTON, ROBERT HOGAN, AND MARY D. SALTER AINSWORTH

The earliest manifestation of obedience in an infant appears in the final quarter of the first year of life. It consists of conforming to such simple maternal commands and prohibitions as "No! No!" and "Come here!" In addition, some infants may occasionally show a self-imposed compliance to prior commands by stopping themselves while approaching a previously prohibited area or reaching for a forbidden object. Some babies heed commands and prohibitions more readily and consistently than others. This study analyzes certain conditions associated with these early manifestations of obedience, and in particular those conditions defined by variations in maternal behavior.

Although infant obedience is a simple behavioral phenomenon, it bears on one of the most fundamental problems in social and developmental psychology, the origins of socialization—those processes which dispose a child to act in accordance with the rules, values, and prescriptions of his society. The excellent reviews which have recently appeared (e.g., Goslin 1969; Zigler

& Child 1968) suggest that two processes, broadly labeled learning and identification, can account for these phenomena. Social learning theory features the learning process and the psychoanalytic tradition features identification. Although the two viewpoints are distinct in many details, they share important assumptions about socialization.

The first assumption is that a child, in the process of being socialized, acquires a set of specific roles, attitudes, and responses that typically conform with social pressures. A child may learn these responses because he has been reinforced for them, or he may imitate the behavior of the person with whom he identifies. Regardless of the process involved, however, it is implied that a child acquires a willingness to comply with specific rules, roles, and response patterns at the same time that he acquires the behaviors themselves. Thus, a distinction is not maintained between the process of learning the values and prescriptions of society and the disposition to comply with them.

It is equally plausible to postulate that the most important step in the socialization process occurs when a child develops a willingness to behave as his elders wish him to. The specific content of parental demands will depend on many factors, including family structure, ethnic heritage, social class, and cultural milieu. Yet, the development of an initial unspecified disposition toward compliance may be critical for the effectiveness of all further socialization practices. If a child lacks this tendency, he may remain in many ways a stranger to his culture, regarding its rules and values from "an external point of view" (Hart 1961).

A second assumption common to both the "learning" and identification" models concerns recognition of the central problem of socialization. The conventional formulation is: "What must be done to a child so that he acts in accordance with the rules of his society?" Such a formulation implies that children who are normally socialized become so only as a result of specific intervention tactics designed to foster social learning or identification. It further implies that the small minority of deviant or unsocialized children have become so because socialization procedures were inadequately applied. The central question might be formulated alternatively as: "What must be done to a child to estrange him from his society?" Such a shift in perspective suggests that socialization is the predictable outcome of development in the "ordinary expectable" social environment; the major practical problem becomes one of preventing or correcting asocial and antisocial behavior in a deviant minority.

The third assumption implied in most treatises on socialization is that there is a fundamental antagonism between a child and his society, between natural behavioral tendencies and cultural constraints. Some writers regard society as inimical to the wholesome development of man's true nature; others consider society as necessarily inhibiting the anarchic natural impulses of the individual for the good of the whole (e.g., Freud 1961). In either case, man and society are conceived to be in essential conflict.

An equally defensible set of assumptions is: man has evolved as a social species; infants are genetically biased toward certain social behaviors; they are preadapted to an ordinary expectable social environment (a social environment similar in essential respects to that in which the species evolved); and thus, children are social from the beginning. Furthermore, adults, especially mothers—despite great cultural and individual variations—are also biased toward responding to infants' signals (Bowlby 1969). Thus, the ordinary expectable social environment for a young child is both responsive and protective. These assumptions imply a fundamental compatibility between man and society, and that societal living has, in general, facilitated the evolution of the human species rather than distorted it (Wallace 1961: 45–83).

The alternative assumptions presented above contain an important common theme: a disposition for obedience—and indeed a disposition to become socialized—tends to develop in children reared in a social environment similar to that in which the species was adapted. The disposition does not require as a condition for its acquisition a rigorous and specialized training regimen. Deviations from the proper environment may produce anomalies in social behavior that other experiences and training cannot change. This theme and the assumptions from which it is derived have the status of theoretical first principles, the value of which ultimately must be determined empirically. Unfortunately, there has been a virtual absence of research directed specifically toward the origins of obedience in infants. The data to be presented below were gathered in the context of another project—the development of an infant's attachment to his mother. These data contain some observations relevant to the concepts presented above regarding the development of obedience.

The specific hypotheses tested in the analysis of these data were that an infant whose mother is accepting, cooperative, and sensitive to signals will tend to obey her verbal commands and prohibitions more consistently than an infant whose mother is rejecting, interfering, and insensitive, and that this tendency to comply is independent of his mother's specific socialization tactics or disciplinary procedures. These hypotheses do not comprehend the entire theoretical corpus sketched above, although they bear on its chief theme, namely that a disposition to comply develops in a social environment which does not deviate unduly from the environment of evolutionary adaptedness, and that such a disposition does not require specific training.

Method

Subjects

The subjects were 25 infant-mother pairs from white middle-class families who were originally contacted through pediatricians in private practice. They were observed at 3-week intervals for 4 hours during home visits throughout the first year of life in conjunction with a longitudinal study of the development of infant-mother attachment, portions of which have been reported elsewhere (Ainsworth & Bell 1969, 1970; Ainsworth, Bell, & Stayton 1971; Ainsworth & Wittig 1969). Of the infants, 15 were boys, 10 were girls. Six of the boys but none of the girls were first born.

Observations, Records, and Assessments

Narrative reports were prepared of the naturalistic observations and interview material obtained during the home visits.

These reports featured detailed play-by-play accounts of infant behavior and relevant maternal activity. For the purposes of this paper only, the reports covering the period from age 9 to 12 months were used.

The following measures were utilized in this analysis:

Maternal variables. Three scales were devised to assess the degree of harmony in the mother-infant interaction: sensitivity-insensitivity, acceptance-rejection, and cooperation-interference. These scales were constructed as 9-point dimensions with the anchor points of 9, 7, 5, 3, and 1 being defined in detail. The behavioral descriptions of the extreme poles will be summarized here.

The sensitive mother is defined as one who is finely attuned to the baby's signals and communications and able to see things from his point of view. She is aware of signals, interprets them accurately, and responds to them promptly and appropriately. The insensitive mother is geared almost exclusively to her own wishes, moods, and activity; her interventions tend to be prompted by signals within herself and therefore are rarely contingent upon the baby's signals.

The acceptance-rejection scale focuses on the balance between a mother's positive and negative feelings about her baby and on the extent to which she has been able to integrate and resolve these conflicting feelings. The accepting mother is judged to accept almost all aspects of the baby's behavior, including those things other mothers find hurtful or distasteful, and she also accepts the responsibility of caring for him without chafing at the temporary restriction of her usual activities. The rejecting mother may have positive feelings about her infant, but they are frequently overwhelmed by resentful and angry feelings which she may voice openly or display less overtly in her behavior toward him and her comments about him.

The cooperative mother avoids imposing her will on the baby but, rather, arranges the environment and her schedule so as to minimize any need to interrupt or to control him. When she intervenes she is adept at "mood setting," which helps him to accept her wishes or controls as something congenial to him. At the other extreme, the interfering mother does not consider her baby as a separate person whose activities and wishes have a validity of their own. She seems to assume that she has a perfect right to do with him what she wishes, imposing her will on his, shaping him to her standards, and interrupting him arbitrarily without regard for his moods, wishes, or activity-in-progress.

Mothers were rated on these three scales by two or more independent judges for each home visit (narrative report) made in the last quarter of the infant's first year. The final rating for each mother was nearly always the median of the visit ratings provided by the judges. The reliability of the ratings is shown by a high level of interjudge agreement. The mean correlation among three judges for acceptance-rejection was .88, and for cooperation-interference .86. Only two judges were compared in the case of sensitivity-insensitivity, and the correlation was .89.

In addition to the three scaled variables, three specific maternal behaviors were coded to assess the extent to which the mother tried to train, discipline, and/or control the baby's behavior. These coded measures were: frequency of verbal commands, frequency of physical intervention, and extent of floor freedom permitted the child. These measures are considered indicative of the kind and amount of maternal control rather than a measure of the quality of the mother-infant interaction.

"Frequency of verbal commands" refers to the mean number of commands and prohibitions issued by the mother per visit. Only commands judged to be comprehensible to a baby were recorded, for example, "No! No!" "Don't touch!" "Come!" "Sit!" "Give it to me!" and the like. Furthermore, only those instances were tallied in which the baby was given an opportunity to comply without physical intervention.

"Frequency of physical intervention" refers to the mean number of discipline-oriented physical interventions by the mother per visit. These include all instances in which the mother forcibly reinforced verbal commands, or, in lieu of verbal commands, tried to force the baby to do as she wished, by dragging him away from a forbidden area, slapping him when he reached for something she did not want him to have, pulling him into a sitting position when he was insisting on standing up and the like.

"Floor freedom" refers to the degree to which a baby was permitted to be free on the floor or in a walker during his waking hours. Two groups were identified: mothers who permitted their babies floor freedom during most of their waking hours were assigned a score of 2; those who confined their babies to playpens most of the time were given a score of 1.

Infant variables. Four infant variables were recorded: sex, IQ, compliance to commands, and internalized controls. IQ was assessed by the Griffiths Scale of Mental Development (Griffiths 1954).

"Compliance to commands" was defined by the percentage of instances in which the baby complied with his mother's verbal commands. Included were cases of compliance after some delay as well as instances of prompt obedience; excluded were instances in which a verbal command was followed by physical intervention so quickly that the baby was not allowed sufficient time to obey.

"Internalized controls" refers to self-inhibiting, self-controlling behavior. Three groups were distinguished according to whether self-inhibition was clearly demonstrated, ambiguous, or never observed. A score of 3 was assigned to infants who, on any occasion, were observed to initiate and then spontaneously arrest any act which had been forbidden or punished in the distant past. A score of 2 was given if the only observed instance of self-inhibition followed within minutes of, but not immediately after, a recent prohibition of the mother's. A score of 1 was assigned to infants who did not manifest self-inhibition on any occasion.

Results

The matrix of intercorrelations among the six maternal measures and the four infant variables is presented in table 19.1. The chief findings are as follows:

First, the three measures which assess the quality of the mother's interaction with her infant—sensitivity-insensitivity, acceptance-rejection, and cooperation-interference—are highly

Table 19.1 Intercorrelations Among Maternal and Infant Variables

Variables	1	2	3	4	5	6	7	8	9
Maternal variables:									
1. Sensitivity-insensitivity	...	...	...	...	...	...	...	...	...
2. Acceptance-rejection	91**	...	...	...	...	...	...	...	...
3. Cooperation-interference	87**	88**	...	...	...	...	...	...	...
4. Verbal commands (frequency)	−14	−05	−35	...	...	...	...	...	...
5. Physical interventions (frequency)	−44*	−38	−59**	62**	...	...	...	...	...
6. Floor freedom (permission of)	07	00	10	−03	07	...	...	...	...
Infant variables:									
7. Sex	−28	−19	−11	−14	17	03	...	...	...
8. IQ	46*	45*	44*	06	06	46*	20	...	...
9. Internalized controls	40*	41*	42*	−15	−27	47*	18	52*	...
10. Compliance to commands	63**	67**	62**	−08	−22	09	−14	38	35

NOTE: Decimals omitted.

* $p < .05$.
** $p < .01$.

intercorrelated. Furthermore, as expected, the infant's compliance to commands is strongly and positively related, to all three indices of the quality of the mother-child relationship.

Second, the two measures of maternal discipline—frequency of verbal commands and frequency of physical interventions—are positively correlated. As hypothesized, however, neither disciplinary practices nor the amount of floor freedom permitted the infant is significantly related to the compliance to commands.

Third, the infant's use of internalized controls is not significantly correlated with compliance to commands. Internalized controls are, however, positively related to IQ, to the amount of floor freedom permitted the baby, and also to maternal sensitivity, acceptance, and cooperation.

Discussion

The findings suggest that a disposition toward obediance emerges in a responsive, accommodating social environment without extensive training, discipline, or other massive attempts to shape the infant's course of development. These findings cannot be predicted from models of socialization which assume that special intervention is necessary to modify the otherwise asocial tendencies of children. Clearly, these findings require a theory that assumes that an infant is initially inclined to be social and (somewhat later) ready to obey those persons who are most significant in his social environment.

Such an alternative viewpoint is offered by the ethological-evolutionary model of early social development presented by Bowlby (1958, 1969) and Ainsworth (1967, 1969). According to this theory, the infant has a species-characteristic repertoire of behaviors that are most readily activated and/or terminated by stimulus conditions provided by adults. These behaviors initially orient an infant to his companions and promote proximity to or contact with them; later they are the modes through which he actively seeks proximity, contact, and social interaction. These proximity-promoting behaviors, which predispose a baby to become attached, are initially indiscriminate as to target, but they gradually focus on that figure who most often interacts with him. Thus, an infant's social behaviors soon become especially directed to his mother (and perhaps a few supplementary figures) and promote attachment and harmonious relations between them.

Through ensuring a certain degree of infant-mother proximity, attachment provides an obvious safeguard against the possible dangers of exploratory behavior. Thus, by protecting the young, attachment bonds promote the survival of populations and/or individuals and account for the "selection" of proximity-promoting behaviors in an evolutionary sense.

Obedience and locomotor exploration appear at about the same time that attachments form. As an infant moves about to investigate his world, his mother must be able to control his actions across an enlarged and often hazardous environment. Thus, it would be biologically advantageous if the development of infant-mother attachment were accompanied by the development of compliance with maternal signals.

Although the ethological literature suggests that the attachment bond disposes an infant to obey his mother's signals, there is little evidence that obedience is achieved through training or specific schedules of reward or punishment. Rather, the affectional tie itself seems to foster a willingness to comply with parental signals.

Most instances of obedience observed in this investigation were acts of simple compliance to present, external signals. "Internalized controls"—self-arrest, self-inhibition—were observed in only 20 percent of our sample, and only in those 1-year-olds who were most accelerated in cognitive development. Although internalized controls were not significantly correlated with simple compliance, they were with the maternal variables of sensitivity, acceptance, and cooperation. It remains for others whose data are not confined to the first year of life to explore adequately the relationships between early compliance and more mature social conduct.

20

And Daddy Makes Three

The Father's Impact on Mother and Young Child

K. ALISON CLARKE-STEWART

The traditional role of the mother is familiar, and the effects of maternal behavior on young children are well-studied, if not well known. But what do we know of the comparable role of the father and of paternal contributions to early development? One review that sought to answer that question summed up the state of our knowledge with the claim that fathers are "forgotten contributors to child development" (Lamb 1975a). Recent publication of a number of books about fathers, both scholarly and popular (e.g., Biller & Meredith 1974; Lamb 1976c; Levine 1977; Lynn 1974), suggests that fathers are no longer forgotten—but the nature of their role and their contribution to children's development remains uncharted and unknown. Careful and systematic observation of children and their fathers is needed if we are to discover how fathers act and affect their families.

Only recently has research focused on paternal behavior. One kind of study of fathers has sought to demonstrate how active and involved they are in child care. The aim of such research seems to be to prove that fathers are as good at parenting as mothers. These studies have shown that fathers are "engrossed" in their infants (Greenberg & Morris 1974) and just as nurturant, affectionate, responsive, and active as mothers (Parke & O'Leary 1976)—at least when interaction is clearly expected and an observer is taking notes. Unfortunately, the distinction between competence and performance limits generalization from these results; although these studies show that fathers can be as active as mothers, they do not establish how much fathers actually do care for their infants in the "privacy of their own homes." Home observations and parental reports (Ban & Lewis 1974; Kotelchuck 1976; Lewis & Weinraub 1974; Pedersen & Robson 1969; Rebelsky & Hanks 1971) suggest that in most homes the opportunities for fathers to display their nurturant talents are not frequent. Estimates of the amount of time fathers spend with their youngsters never exceed 3 hours per day—often they are considerably less—and the amount of father-child interaction actually observed has been far, far less.

The alternative approach to demonstrating how much fathers are like mothers has been to investigate how different they are. This approach has also been followed in recent work. Differences between men's and women's responses to children have been documented (e.g., Berman 1976), and the difference in biological "connectedness" of mothers and fathers to their offspring has been noted (e.g., Lewis & Weinraub 1976). It has been suggested that because of the biological link between mother and infants the mother's role is more likely to involve physical caregiving, while the father's role involves fun and games and a link to the outside world (Lamb 1975a; Lewis & Weinraub 1976). Few observational data demonstrating such differences in parental styles of interaction have been collected as yet, however.

Differences in children's behavior to mother and father have also been interpreted in the context of children's social development, particularly the development of attachment. The consensus of recent research on this issue (see review by Parke 1978) seems to be that attachment to the mother, while undeniably special, is not unique. In terms of physical proximity and contact or reactions to separation, children form attachments to both parents, although for children under 2 years mother is usually the preferred target.

In recent discussions of children's relations with their parents, these proximal attachment behaviors have been separated from the distal or "affiliative" social behaviors of looking, talking, smiling, and playing. In contrast to the prevalent finding that attachment, when differential, favors the mother, it has been suggested that affiliative behavior favors the father—that children actually prefer the father, because fathers are "simply more fun to interact with" (Lamb 1976c:6).

The explicit, though as yet unsupported, supposition of researchers demonstrating differences in parents' or children's behavior is that mothers and fathers have different influences on children's development (e.g., Lamb 1977a). Research to support this supposition by correlating maternal and paternal variables with assessments of the child's development in the first few years, unfortunately, is not common. Too often, investigations of paternal predictors of development have focused only on the father-child relation and ignored the concurrent contribution of the mother (e.g., Epstein & Radin 1975; Radin 1973). This exclusive concentration on the father is as shortsighted as the previously popular exclusive research focus on mothers. To fully understand parental correlates of children's development, it is necessary to examine relations with both mother and father simultaneously, to consider the family as a triadic system. This suggests a research approach that gives attention to all the possible relations within the family, looking for indirect as well as direct effects of parental attitudes and behavior on children's development.

Such an approach was followed in the present study by examining relations between behaviors of mother and child, father and child, and mother and father. In addition, the investigation integrated these triadic relations with data on differences in children's attachment and affiliation to mother and father and in mothers' and fathers' attitudes and interaction with children. Furthermore, it examined the interactive patterns among mother, father, and child as they changed developmentally over time.

Method

Data were collected in a longitudinal study of 14 children carried out in 1972–1973. They were all white, but included various socioeconomic levels: six families could be categorized as working class, five as middle class, and three as professional class. All fathers were employed full time; all mothers were nonworking and their children's primary caregivers. There were seven boys and seven girls in the study, all first or second born. Data were gathered in different ways: unstructured "natural" observations, semistructured "probe" situations, and standardized developmental tests.

Natural Observations

Six 1-hour observations were made of the children as they behaved naturally and spontaneously at home: three when both mother and father were home, and three when mother was the only parent present. The visits occurred when the children were approximately 15, 20, and 30 months of age, ages selected to both overlap (15–20 months) and extend (30 months) previous research on father-child interactions.

Before the observation, parents were instructed to ignore the observer and go about their normal activities as far as possible while the observer followed and recorded the activities of the child. The observational record was marked in 10-second intervals at the sound of a beeper in the observer's ear, and any behavior was recorded only once during a 10-second period (unless it was interrupted by another behavior and then resumed). Each behavior was indexed as "R" (responsive) which it occurred in direct response to the behavior of the other person.

Semistructured Situations

Assessment of attachment. After the natural observations at the two visits when the children were 20 months of age, children's attachment to each parent was measured. An identical procedure was followed by the mother at one visit (when the father was not present) and by the father at the other visit (when the mother was in the house but not in the room). It consisted of the following steps: the parent sat at some distance from the child and ignored him for 1 min, then looked, smiled, and talked to him for 1 min, called him to come (1 min), engaged him in social interaction (2 min), and played with him using a book (4 min); then the parent left the child (1 min), left the child's room (2 min), returned (1 min), left the house (2 min), and returned once more (1 min). The observer, meanwhile, recorded on a checklist for each step of the sequence the child's behavior to the parent (looking at and away, smiling, frowning, vocalizing, gesturing, fretting, crying, touching, affectionately touching, clinging, approaching, avoiding, and staying close or distant).

Play probes. Two parallel "play probes" were carried out following the hour of natural observation at the two consecutive home visits when the children were 30 months old: the first with mother and child only, the second with father, mother, and child. Parents were asked on these occasions to involve the child in a variety of specific play activities: dyadic activities (e.g., blowing bubbles, making designs with drinking straws, playing with a toy telephone, reading a book) or triadic activities (playing a game, coloring, throwing or rolling a ball). Before each dyadic play activity in the second probe when mother and father were both present, the child was asked which parent he wanted to do the particular activity with, and that parent played first; then, after a specified length of time, the experimenter asked the child to do the activity with the other parent, and that parent continued the activity for an identical length of time.

Developmental Assessments

Finally, one further kind of data was analyzed for the present report: assessment of the child's intellectual competence. The Bayley Mental Development Scale was administered by a trained tester at the university to each child at 16 months and again at

22 months. As some of the subjects had already reached the ceiling on the Bayley Mental Scale at 22 months, for the third time period the Minnesota Child Development Inventory (MCDI) was completed by the child's mother. This last test yielded a composite score based largely on conceptual ability and language comprehension and production, and was roughly comparable to the Bayley Scale. Since intellectual competence measures were neither collected by nor available to the home observers, these developmental assessments were independent of the data on parents.

Results

Children's Behavior to Mother and Father

The first analysis of these data was the comparison of children's behavior with their mothers and fathers.

The semistructured assessment of children's attachment to mother and father offered results that were clear and consistent. When parents' behaviors were specified and controlled in these interaction and separation episodes at 20 months, no measure of attachment behavior differentiated children's relations with mother and father. This was true for measures of proximity and contact prior to separation, for measures of reaction to separation and reunion, and appeared in both quantified indices of distress and pleasure and observers' overall rating of attachment. Nor was a difference observed in the amount of affiliative interaction (smiling, vocalizing, and playing) with mother versus father in this situation. Only one measure differentiated children's reactions to mother and father in the attachment assessment: children were rated significantly more responsive to play initiated by father than play initiated by mother.

This positive reaction to play with the father was even more clearly differentiated from the reaction to play with mother 10 months later, when children played with both parents in the triadic play probe. Eight of the 14 consistently chose to play with father first and displayed a stronger preference for him as playmate.

This "preference" for play with the father is based on differential quality of play, not quantity, and occurred when parents or children were requested to so interact. In the natural observation, by contrast, in which the amount or frequency of interaction was assessed and no request for play was made, mother was clearly the predominant partner.

Differences and Similarities between Mothers and Fathers

During the hours that fathers were at home for the natural observation, mothers were observed to interact more with the children than fathers did, not only in overall amount—touches, $F(1,12) = 21.74$, $p < .001$; verbal, $F(1,12) = 25.09$, $p < .001$; negative, $F(1,12) = 11.03$, $p < .01$; plays object, $F(1,12) = 7.59$, $p < .01$—but as a proportion of their time together—verbal/in room, $F(1,9) = 6.02$, $p < .05$.

Effect of the Father on Mother-child Interaction

For all the results described thus far, the data were limited to situations in which mother and father were both present. The possibility that the mother's behavior was affected by the father's presence was explored by comparing maternal behavior in matched pairs of father present–father absent observations. From these analyses of variance it appeared that there was a significant effect on the mother's behavior in having the father in the house: the amount of positive and responsive talk by the mother to the infant when father was home was significantly less.

But merely being "at home" is not the best measure of the father's presence. We therefore analyzed separately "in room" behavior in those observations during which father was not only at home but in the same room as mother and child for more than two-thirds of the observation period (23 observations). When father was in the room, mother talked, responded, and played with the child less.

Parents' Behavior and Child Development

Finally, analyses were carried out to examine associations of maternal and paternal behavior with children's development. This was accomplished by correlating parental variables with measures of children's intellectual ability (Bayley Mental Scale at 16 and 22 months and the MCDI at 30 months).

For maternal variables, children's intellectual competence was most highly and consistently (on more than one IQ measure) related to the mother's verbal and materials stimulation, intellectual acceleration, and expression of warmth and positive emotion; it was not related to her physical contact, time in the same room, or amount of play. The patterns for fathers, however, were somewhat different. The paternal variables most closely associated with children's intelligence were the father's engagement of the child in play in the probe ($r = .50, p < .06$), his positive ratings of the child ($r = .74, p < .01$), his anticipation of the child's independence, and the duration of his interactions with the child in the natural observations ($r = .50, p < .06$).

The final analysis of these data was the examination of changes in parent-child correlations over time. Differences had been documented in the patterns of associations of maternal and paternal behavior with child development; were there also differences in the directions of those associations? By calculating and comparing the cross-lagged correlations for parental and child behaviors at two time periods, it has been suggested, the most plausible direction of influence between parents' and children's behavior can be inferred (see procedure in Clarke-Stewart 1973). This manipulation was performed on a set of parental variables and child measures from the present study. Three parental variables were selected for this statistical treatment to illustrate the three central kinds of parent-child interaction discussed in this article: verbal interaction, social play, and object play. These were correlated with assessments of the child's intellectual development that were made within a month of the observation (at 15 and 30 months).

In the results of the cross-lagged correlational analysis, too, a consistent difference between mothers and fathers was apparent. The predominant direction of association for mother-child variables was from mother at time 1 to child at time 2. That is, the mothers' verbal stimulation and play with toys at 15 months were more closely related to children's intellectual performance at 30 months (for boys, r's = .63 and .61; for girls, r's = .58 and .30) than was children's intellectual performance at 15 months related to maternal verbalization and play at 30 months (for boys, r's = .10 and .04; for girls, r's = .18 and .24). For fathers, the pattern of correlations was in the opposite direction; that is, children's intellectual performance at 15 months was associated with subsequent paternal talk and play 15 months later (r's = .81 vs. .16 and .38 vs. −.08 for girls' talk and play, and .33 vs. −.03 for boys' play).

One further analysis completed the treatment of data in the present study. Cross-lagged correlations between the mothers' and fathers' behavior were also examined for the same three variables. The findings from this analysis showed the father's talking and playing with the child at one age to be highly associated with the mother's talking and play with the child later (r's from .55 to .89 compared with r's from .06 to .34).

Discussion

While strong empirical conclusions based on this study alone are impossible because of the small sample size and exploratory nature of the investigation, the results offered merit discussion. Simplest to deal with is the study's confirmation of previous research showing that children's proximal-attachment behavior with mother and father is highly similar.

More controversial are the results relating to the affiliative preference for fathers that has been postulated by Lamb (1976b, 1976c, 1976d, 1977a; Lamb 1975b). In the present study, children were observed to enjoy and cooperate more in play with their fathers than with their mothers. At issue, however, is whether the difference thus observed offers evidence that children prefer their fathers or merely that they are responding to a more engaging play style on the father's part. The weight of evidence, from the present study—and Lamb's—seems to point to the latter explanation and to suggest that the concept of preference is inaccurate and may be misleading. It seems most likely, then, that differences in the amount of children's affiliative behavior are a function of parental behavior. Only when fathers play, apparently, does children's preferential reaction appear.

The question this raises, then, is, What is the play style that fathers adopt? The present study suggests it is a style that the parent also enjoys, one which involves praise for the child and social-physical rather than intellectual activities or interaction with objects; it occurs in briefer rather than in extended episodes, and it may also be associated with negative affect from the parent (those fathers who played most were most negative to the child). These findings corroborate the results of other investigators who have noted the physical and physically stimulating, rough-and-tumble, nonintellectual nature of paternal play (Lamb 1976c, 1977b; Lynn & Cross 1974; Parke & O'Leary 1976; Pedersen & Robson 1969; Lamb 1975b, 1977c; Yogman 1977; Lamb 1975c).

The reason this particular style is more common for fathers than for mothers has yet to be established; we do not know whether it is a function of biological sex differences, cultural expectations, or merely the extent of relative experience mothers and fathers have with (their) children. This question is one that should be explored empirically.

In highlighting the differences between mothers' and fathers' play styles and roles, it is important to place these differences in the broader context of all the observed differences and similarities between mothers and fathers. In natural observations, mothers were observed to be more interactive than fathers in amounts of verbalization, physical contact, and play with toys; but they were not different from fathers in measures of responsiveness, stimulatingness, affection, or effectiveness, or in the patterns of intercorrelations among their behaviors (except, as mentioned, for social play). The simplest generalization to draw from these results seems to be that mothers and fathers are unlike in quantity of interaction with their children but alike in its quality—with the one notable exception of social play, where they are alike in quantity but unlike in quality.

A complication is added to observations of parent-child interaction when the interaction occurs in dyadic versus triadic situations. In the present study, when both parents were present, mothers initiated less talk and play with the children than when they were alone with them. This finding illustrates the more general phenomenon that, as the number of adults in a situation increases, the amount of adult-child interaction decreases, since adults concentrate more on each other (Lamb 1976a; Lamb 1977d; Cleaves & Rosenblatt 1977).

Further evidence for indirect versus direct contributions to child development in the present study is provided by analyses of correlations between parental variables and assessments of children's intellectual competence. Patterns of correlations obtained in these analyses suggest that maternal variables associated with intellectual performance, by virtue of their acceleratory and stimulating nature (verbal and materials stimulation and intellectual acceleration), are likely to be influences on the child's intellectual development, while the paternal variables most closely associated with children's intellectual competence (expecting early independence, being able to engage the child in play, rating the child high on competence, and interacting with the child longer) are more likely to be the result of the child's competence. Cross-lagged and partial correlational analyses of parent and child variables over time support this view, suggesting that the most plausible causal direction—if such can be inferred—is mother influencing child, child influencing father, and father infuencing mother, over the time period assessed.

The hypothesis that the mother's effect on child development is direct and the father's indirect, supported by this preliminary evidence, appears to be one that merits further exploration. The suggestion from this study of a triadic chain of influence in the family from mother to child to father to mother, while fascinating, is highly tentative. It is based on a small sample of relatively "traditional" families and relates only to children's intellectual development, to parents' verbal and playful interaction, and to the age period from 15 to 30 months. Its particular usefulness is to illustrate the complexity of parent-child relations.

21

Mother, Father, and Infant as an Interactive System

FRANK A. PEDERSEN

Recent research on fathers and infants represents a healthy recognition that the sum total of the infant's early environmental experience is not simply limited to the infant's relationship with the mother. On the other hand, if this new research emphasis is concentrated solely on the father-infant relationship without regard for the mother-infant unit, it will be as shortsighted as the past emphasis upon mother and infant alone. The proposition addressed here is that the family unit of mother, father, and infant represents an interactive network, with each family member influencing and being influenced by the other members. One particular vantage point will be the father because there is a dearth of conceptualization regarding the father in the infancy period, but similar ideas may be developed from the vantage point of the mother or infant.

The basic assumption behind our research endeavor was that the mother-infant interaction does not occur in a psychological vacuum, even though much research appears to assume that it does. Within the middle-class nuclear family, the father is a potent psychological force whose behavior affects and is affected by both mother and infant. This occurs in two ways: by the father's relationship with the infant and by his relationship with the mother.

His interaction with the infant may have important consequences for development. One of the stereotypes of our culture is that fathers often engage in frolicsome "horse-play" with babies. A father may vigorously bounce an infant and lift it overhead. It is common to see infants respond with peals of laughter and occasionally a twinge of apprehensiveness. We can hypothesize that frequent play of this nature may encourage the infant to become more receptive to activities involving rapid rates of stimulus change, an experience which might in turn enhance the development of exploratory behavior. The infant may develop an expectancy for robust play from his father, and the father whose child enjoys this type of play would be reinforced for his involvement and is likely to provide more of these experiences.

It is also likely that the father's relationship with the infant has consequences for the mother as well. How the father interacts—or does not interact—with the infant may affect the experiences the mother provides for the infant. In other words, the father's behavior may have a secondary impact that is mediated by the mother. In the terminology of Bronfenbrenner (1974), this is a "second order effect." The father's involvement in caregiving activities may provide a respite which is supportive to the mother. There also can be a subtle or very direct transmission of his feelings about the infant and his child-rearing values. If the father feels positively towards the infant, it is likely that the mother's positive feelings and behaviors will be supported and enhanced. If the father is impatient with babies, short-tempered about their fussing, or interacts in a style with which the mother is uncomfortable, this may have an unsettling effect on the mother, and she may feel the need to buffer or compensate for the father's feelings and behavior.

The father may affect the mother in a second way. The husband-wife relationship may influence the quality of the mother's behavior with the infant. A warm, affectionate husband-wife relationship may support the mother by meeting her dependency needs, and she may then find it easier to express nurturant behavior towards the child. On the other hand, if the husband-wife relationship is distant or characterized by tension and conflict, the thwarting of the mother's needs for intimacy may foster reactivity to the affectional needs of her baby. She may develop a very close relationship with the infant as compensation for what is lacking in the relationship with her husband, or she may show negative affect or irritability, a displacement of her own feelings in regard to her husband.

The bidirectional nature of these relationships should be underscored. An infant's special sensitivities and responsiveness to certain types of stimulation may "turn on" either parent in very selective ways. A "difficult baby," that is, one who is particularly fussy, irritable, or hard to soothe, may be a trying experience for both parents, and a variety of conflicts and disagreements may arise between the parents over what is the most appropriate way of responding to the infant. Similarly, the father's behavior with the infant is also influenced by the mother; her behavior and feelings toward the infant and their relationship with each other may impinge upon his handling of the child.

Having sketched out examples of these complex sets of bidirectional relationships, selected data will be presented which bear on whether these ideas are merely figments of my imagination.

Method

The data come from a sample of 39 first-born infants (20 males and 19 females) and their parents, participants in a larger investigation carried out in the Social and Behavioral Sciences Branch of the National Institute of Child Health and Human Development (NICHD). Fathers ranged in age from 18 to 36, with a mean age of 26 years. Mothers' ages ranged from 18 to 36, with a mean age of 25 years. All families were nonminority and middle class, recruited during the last trimester of pregnancy through the National Naval Medical Center in Bethesda and private obstetricians. Only normal infants free of complications of pregnancy, labor, and delivery were included. Apgar scores were all normal. Almost half of the parents in the sample had attended Lamaze classes in natural childbirth.

For the analyses which will be reported, there were three

sources of data:

1. *Neonatal Behavioral Assessment*. Between 42 and 72 hours after birth, the infants were examined in the hospital nursery with the Neonatal Behavioral Assessment Scales (Brazelton 1973) by a trained examiner. Through factor analysis and conceptual considerations, a number of items were combined into 3 clusters. These clusters, which accounted for 13 items of the examination, were the following: (1) Alertness (responsivity to various stimuli), (2) Irritability (the frequency and conditions of state changes and fussing behaviors), and (3) Motor Maturity (smoothness of the baby's movements and absence of tremulousness and startling). Similar clusters have been identified by other investigators, e.g., Tronick and Brazelton (1975).

2. *Mother-Infant Relationship*. Ratings were made of the quality of the mother-infant relationship in connection with two time-sampling home observations when the infants were 4 weeks old. Among these seven variables, each of which was a five-point rating scale summed for the two observations, one was selected out because of its pivotal relationships with the other sets of data. That rating was Feeding Competence, and refers to the appropriateness of the mother in managing feeding. Mothers rated high were judged able to pace the feeding well, intersperse feeding and efforts to relieve ingested air without disrupting the baby, and seemed sensitive to the baby's needs for either stimulation of feeding or brief rest periods during the course of feedings. Each hour-long observation included a feeding, and since the babies were only 4 weeks old, that event tended to dominate the observation. Adequate interobserver agreement was established between pairs of observers with 10 cases not in the main data sample.

3. *Father-Infant and Husband-Wife Relationships*. The third source of data was interviews with the fathers, conducted by a male psychiatrist in our laboratory when the infants were from 4 to 5 weeks old. For these analyses, two areas were of particular interest: each father's report of his relationship with the infant, and his description of the husband-wife relationship. The father described how much he played with his baby, whether and how often he engaged in caregiving activities such as feeding and

changing diapers, and he described his affective reactions to his baby. He also described his relationship with his wife, whether he felt supportive toward her, whether he evaluated her maternal behavior in positive terms, and whether there was an appreciable amount of tension, conflict, and disagreement in their marital relationship. Five ratings entered into these analyses and each variable summarized responses to several questions in the respective areas. Inter-rater agreement was established with independent judgements made by a psychologist based on tape recordings of 10 interviews. Product-moment correlations between ratings exceeded .85 for all variables.

There was absolute methodological independence in these three sets of measures. Staff members involved with one set had no knowledge of either of the other two. Moreover, there was total situational independence in the data collection. Fathers were not present when mothers were observed, mothers were not present during the father interviews, and neither parent observed the Brazelton. In the case of the father interviews, however, both the father-infant and husband-wife relationships were appraised, so these content areas are not methodologically independent. Establishing relationships among the three sets of measures therefore means that relatively enduring linkages may exist. The data must be sensitive to something more than merely situational consistencies or consistencies based on the cognitive construction of parents which are not independently ascertainable.

Results and Discussion

The analyses were based on product-moment correlations among variables from the three data sets, which utilize a total of nine measures. Male and female infants were analyzed separately. For the female infants, there were few conceptually meaningful relationships. In the sample of male infants, however, several significant relationships were found, which for the most part were supportive of the conceptual formulation that was proposed.

Figure 21.1 reports the network of correlations for male infants.

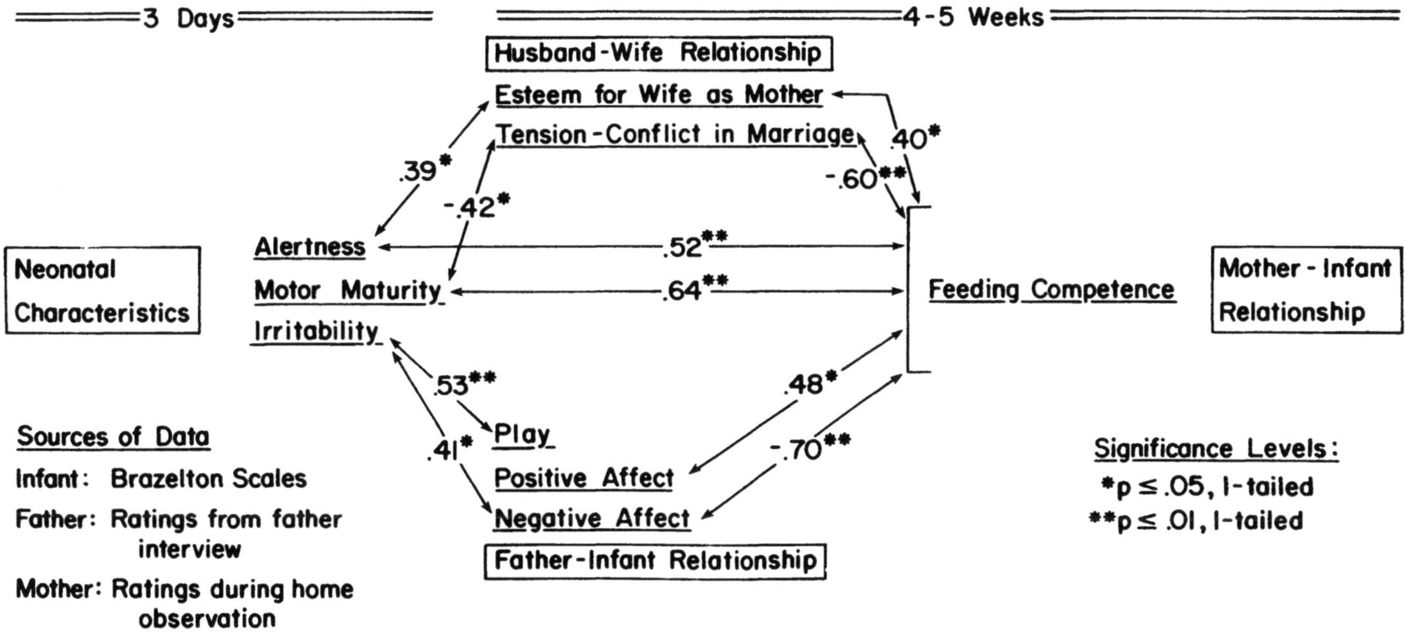

Figure 21.1 Selected Variables Illustrating Mother-Father-Infant Interrelationships (Male Infants N = 20).

Each arrow represents a significant relationship. The absence of an arrow between two variables in different sets means that a correlation was not significant. In understanding the results, two caveats must be considered from the outset. First, the data are all correlational. This means that the *direction* of influence is indeterminate. Second, as in all correlational investigations, a statistically significant relationship between two measures may be causally associated with other variables, ones that were not fully appraised in this investigation. Therefore, it would appear prudent to view these results as merely providing a basis for developing hypotheses of psychological linkages among different family members.

Figure 21.1 indicates that neonatal characteristics, assessed at 3 days of age, were related to subsequent mother-infant and father-infant interaction, as well as to the husband-wife relationship. Because of the temporal order of these assessments, there is a strong temptation to view the results as an "infant effect" in the manner that Bell (1968) has proposed. From what is known of the larger investigation, however, this view would be simplistic. Other analyses (Standley et al. 1978) indicated that neonatal behavior assessed with the Brazelton scales was sensitive to maternal medication during the delivery. Medication, of course, is not randomly administered, but is influenced by the mother's personality, the physician's clinical judgment, and the type of childbirth experience the family desires. The latter may be influenced by participation in a childbirth preparation group, which may have important implications for the husband-wife relationship during the pregnancy and the delivery itself. In short, it is likely that the correlations are best understood as tapping into an ongoing process of reciprocal influence and feedback which was underway before the birth of the baby.

Figure 21.1 indicates that the infant's alertness and motor maturity are associated with qualities of the marital relationship. With higher levels of infant alertness, the father evaluated the mother more positively in her performance of nurturant behaviors. In families where babies showed higher levels of motor maturity, there was a significant tendency for the marital relationship to be characterized by lower levels of tension and conflict. Stated more boldly, a good baby and a good marriage seemed to go together. These relationships extended the anecdotal finding of Leifer and her colleagues (Leifer et al. 1972) into the normal range of infant characteristics and marital disharmony. They found that in families where there was a premature infant, many of whom were presumably at risk for neurological damage, there was a disproportionate number of divorces in the follow-up period compared to the full-term control group. In the present investigation, normal variation in the infant was associated with the marital relationship in intact families. Similarly, these findings are consistent with others based solely on parental report. Russell (1974) found that positive characterizations of the infant were made in families that experienced a more optimal transition to parenthood. In all of these investigations, it is at least theoretically possible that postive aspects of the husband-wife relationship during pregnancy may have contributed to more optimal infant status at birth, or that the infant's neonatal condition may have supported and reinforced marital functioning, or that both areas were mediated by other factors.

The husband-wife relationship was also linked to the mother-infant unit. When the father was more supportive of the mother, that is, when he evaluated her maternal skills more positively, she was more effective in feeding the baby. A psychologically similar pattern was found for marital discord. High tension and conflict in the marriage was associated with more inept feeding on the part of the mother. On the one hand, these associations may be seen as evidence that the marital relationship is a source of social support for the mother and contributes toward more optimal nurturing of the infant. Conversely, the findings may be interpreted in the reverse direction: competent mothers may elicit more positive evaluations from their husbands, and the mother's difficulties in nurturing the infant may impose strain upon the husband-wife relationship. To complete the picture, it is apparent that the infant's alertness and motor maturity are also positively associated with maternal feeding competence. The overall network of relationships is that of a circular system of reciprocal feedback. The systemic nature of relationships is prominent, but correlational data prevent one from assigning an ultimate causative effect to a particular variable.

Irritability in the baby showed quite a different pattern of relationships. Fathers played more with irritable babies, perhaps to distract them in their fussy periods. Social play at age 4 weeks tends to be far less complex than at older ages. Play may be thought of as primarily attentiveness in other than caregiving activities. The fathers were, however, rather reactive in a negative way to the baby's irritability. With higher infant irritability, fathers tended to show more negative affect. The mother's feeding skill was unrelated to how irritable her child was, but there appeared to be an indirect effect of the baby's irritability through the father. When the father described that he felt more negative affect toward the baby, the mother was rated as having more difficulty in feeding. Perhaps she was projecting feelings about her husband qua father into her relationship with her baby and was more anxious and uncertain as a consequence. Infant irritability was not significantly related to the husband-wife relationship in the way that infant alertness and motor maturity were. Instead, the father's route of connectedness with the mother-infant relationship was through his parental behavior.

The general failure to find systematic relations among variables for female infants is both perplexing and disconcerting. It gives little assurance to this effort at theory building. But explanations, like hope, spring eternal. One possibility is that, insofar as neonatal behaviors are a major controlling influence on the total pattern of relationships, then the data in this investigation are not inconsistent with those of Yang and Moss (1978). They found greater longitudinal stability of behavior from the neonatal period for boys than for girls. A second explanation may relate to the high value placed upon male offspring within our culture. Many parents in this investigation were explicit in preferring a male child, and the early adaptations of parents who had their wishes confirmed may express itself in tighter psychological connectedness among mother, father, and infant. This line of reasoning suggests that, with female infants, family members are somewhat more insulated from each other's influence during the early adaptation period.

Because of the variety of issues which may be important in different families, research of this nature is fraught with difficulties. It is important to deal with the idiosyncratic *match* among the qualities of each family member. It may be wrong to prescribe uniformly that high involvement of the father with the infant is an unequivocal benefit in all families. In some families, the father's relationship with his infant may be psychologically threatening to the mother, either because of her insecurity about her maternal skills or the competitive posture with which the father expresses his interest in the infant. In other families the mother may genuinely welcome the father's interest in the infant but she may find that their values and philosophies of child care are radically different and become a source of conflict.

Since how well a family functions is partly determined by the idiosyncratic match among each family member, it is very difficult to develop variables which generalize across families. Variables which differentiate families meaningfully are likely to be rather abstract just so they can transcend the concrete issues of a particular family. The more abstract a concept is, of course, the harder it is to tie it to specific behavioral referents. A related problem is that we must have concepts which characterize dyads or three-person units, while much of psychology deals with individual behavior.

There is a final implication that bears mentioning. Much developmental research has focused on finding antecedent-consequent relations while considering a dyadic unit, usually mother and child but more recently, father and child. When it is clear that a third person is psychologically a part of the influence pathways, such outcome-oriented research has a naïve quality. Statistical relationships between two individuals may be mediated or masked in some indeterminate way by the third. Even in an experimental intervention, with families randomly assigned to different treatment conditions, changing the behavior of one parent may inadvertently alter the behavior of the other in a way that confuses or confounds the effects of the experimental manipulation. It seems desirable to concentrate research resources on understanding the *processes* of family interaction with young infants. Only when more is known about the networks of reciprocal influence can we approach the problem of antecedent-consequent relations with enough understanding to do justice to the task.

22

Interactions Between 18-Month-Olds and Their Preschool Siblings

MICHAEL E. LAMB

In recent years there has been a growing recognition that the infant social world is far more extensive than traditional formulations proposed. Researchers have demonstrated that most infants are attached to both their mothers and fathers from the time they are first capable of forming relationships (Kotelchuck 1976; Lamb 1976c, 1977a) and that infants play an active role in the initiation, modulation, and termination of social interaction (Lamb 1977e). As a result, researchers have begun to examine the infant's ability or willingness to interact with extrafamilial others, such as peers (Eckerman, Whatley, & Kutz 1975; Lewis & Rosenblum 1975; Rubenstein & Howes 1976; Lee 1973). With one exception, however, no attempts have been made to explore the nature of sibling-infant relations. This neglect is surprising, since there is considerable speculation about the role siblings play in socialization (see Sutton-Smith & Rosenberg 1970). In addition, those who have investigated peer relations among infants have found that parents seldom provide their offspring with the opportunity to interact with peers (Lewis et al. 1975). Consequently, interactions with siblings may comprise the bulk of the interaction infants have with other children. The major goal of the present study, therefore, was to investigate the nature and extent of sibling-infant interaction.

We chose to conduct this initial investigation of sibling-infant interaction in a laboratory setting, both to ensure that all sibling pairs were observed in similar social and physical environs and to avoid the disruption of interaction that is likely to occur when two observers (at least) toting intriguing recording devices are readily visible (as they would be in the home). Needless to say, our understanding of sibling-infant relations and their importance will be incomplete until we are able to observe siblings in a variety of differing situations—including the home environment.

In sum, the present study was designed to provide detailed information about the nature and extent of sibling-infant interaction, and to investigate the relative attractiveness of parents and siblings as interaction partners.

Method

Subjects. Twenty-four mother-father/infant groups participated in this study. The infants were all 18 months of age at the time of observation; their siblings were all of preschool age (range 38–70 months; $\overline{X}$ = 53 months). Half of the infants and siblings were boys, half were girls. There were six male infants with older brothers and six with older sisters, as well as six females with older sisters and six with brothers. Subjects were recruited from birth announcements in the local newspaper; 65 percent of the eligible families contacted agreed to participate. Most (75 percent) of the fathers had professional or managerial occupations.

Each sibling-infant dyad was observed for 24 minutes: eight with their mother present, eight with their father, and eight with both parents. The sequence of episodes was varied systematically so that four pairs (one from each of the sex of infant x sex of sibling permutations) were observed in each of the six possible sequences. The parents were instructed to be responsive to the children's initiatives but to refrain from initiating interaction with or between the children.

From behind one-way windows that extended across the length of one wall, two observers each recorded the behavior of one of the children while a third person made a videotape record. The observers were required to record the interaction which their target child had with its parents as well as with its siblings, using the combined observation categories of Eckerman, Whatley, & Kutz (1975) and Lamb (1976c, 1977b). Eckerman, Whatley, & Kutz's definitions of strike, imitate, coordinate play, struggle, same play materials, accept toy, take toy, and take over toy, and Lamb's of smile, vocalize, look (modified), laugh, proffer, proximity, touch, approach, seek to be held, fuss, and adult vocalization were used.

Results

Interaction between siblings. A 2 (age of child: infant or older) × 2 (sex of child) multivariate analysis of variance (MANOVA) of the 13 variables listed in the upper portion of table 22.1 revealed a highly significant effect for age of child, $F(13,128) = 10.33$, $p < .001$, and significant univariate effects on 8 of the measures. Inspection of table 22.1 suggests that the older children were more likely to vocalize or proffer toys to the infants, who were in turn more likely to monitor the others' activity (by watching and maintaining/attaining proximity) and attempt to repeat what they were doing (by imitating and taking over toys). Further analysis of the look variable yielded results consistent with this. The babies were significantly more likely to watch the sibling's actions than to look at the sibling directly; by contrast, the older children were more likely to look at the sibling directly than to look at what s/he was doing (p's $< .01$).

Choice of parent or sibling as interactive partner. To investigate the relative preferences of the children for interaction with parents or siblings, we combined data concerning the two children in a 2 (target: parent or sibling) × 2 (actor: infant or older) MANOVA including as variables the 10 measures which were recorded in coding interaction with both parents and siblings. We found a strong target effect, $F(10,323) > 70$, $p < .0001$.

Table 22.1 Mean Frequency of Interactive Behaviors Per Episode: Sibling Interaction

Behavior	Baby to Older	Older to Baby	Significance of Difference
Smile	.68	1.02	N.S.
Vocalize	1.64	5.64	p < .0001
Look	4.90	2.49	p < .0001
Look at other's activities	6.57	1.64	p < .0001
Laugh	.51	.60	N.S.
Proffer	.22	.58	p < .015
Approach	3.97	2.19	p < .0002
Fuss	.46	.00	N.S.
Strike	.19	.24	N.S.
Imitate	.76	.04	p < .0002
Accept toy	.15	.04	p < .066
Take over toy	1.03	.25	p < .0001
Take toy	.26	.39	N.S.
All measures[a]	21.5	.14	p < .0001
Behaviors Requiring Mutual Participation			
Proximity[b]		132.5	
Touch[b]		.78	
Same play materials		2.91	
Struggle		.58	
Coordinate play		.58	

[a] MANOVA comparison.
[b] Duration measures. Figures refer to mean number of seconds.

Clearly, the children engaged in far more interaction with their parents than with their siblings, though they were likely to be in the proximity of their siblings. Additional analyses revealed that this effect described the preferences of the older and younger children equally well. On only one measure did they differ: The infants looked at their siblings more often than at their parents ($p < .001$), while the older children looked at their parents more often ($p < .004$).

The actor effect was also highly significant ($p < .0001$). While the older siblings were more likely to vocalize in interaction, the infants were significantly more likely to display most other behaviors. Stated differently, the preschoolers were markedly less interested than were the infants in social interaction with either their parents or their siblings. Infants, by contrast, engaged in extensive interpersonal interaction despite (perhaps because of) the novel and varied environment.

A highly significant ($p < .0001$) actor × target interaction indicated that whereas both infants and older children tended to interact with their parents rather than with their siblings, the infants' preferences were more strongly expressed than those of their older siblings. Univariate analyses showed significant effects on the measures vocalize, look, and proffer ($.005 < p$'s $< .0001$), and near-significant effects on tough and fuss (p's $<$ .10).

Discussion

The descriptive analysis of the interaction between siblings revealed that there was surprisingly little direct interaction and an interesting though readily interpretable asymmetry between the roles played by the older and younger children. The preschoolers were more likely than the infants to direct affiliative behaviors to their siblings (by vocalizing or offering toys). The younger children, by contrast, appeared to monitor the whereabouts and activities of their brothers and sisters and took the major role in maintaining proximity between them. Presumably, they learn from trying to employ the toy or repeat the behavior shortly after the (more competent) sibling has done so. Although the infants and older siblings fairly frequently played with the same play materials, these encounters seldom developed into bouts of interactive play.

There are two important conclusions that can be drawn from these data. First, it is clear that the absolute levels of sibling interaction—in the laboratory context (this study) as well as in American (White & Watts 1973) and Kenyan (Edwards & Whiting 1976) homes—are relatively low. In all contexts, it appears that infants prefer to interact with their parents rather than with their siblings when they have the choice. Second, however, it seems that the types of interaction one observes within parent-infant and sibling-infant dyads differ substantially. More specifically, the data reported by Edwards and Whiting (1976) on mother-infant and sibling-infant relations, by Rubenstein and Howes (1976) on peer relations, by Lamb (1977a) on mother- and father-infant play, and those gathered in the present study together suggest that siblings and familiar peers facilitate toy encounters and associated experiences in a way that parents seldom do. Parent-infant play, as Lamb (1977b) reported, is usually directed by the parents and typically occurs at their convenience and upon their initiative. In sibling encounters, by contrast, we seldom see the older children attempting to play with their infant siblings, yet the latter are keenly aware of the preschoolers' behavior, attempt to keep close to them, and often follow the siblings' behavior with attempts to act upon the same toy or imitate the siblings' behavior. Interestingly, Rubenstein and Howes (1976) found that the presence of a familiar peer facilitated the toy play of young infants, and our pilot observations of 12-month-old infants observed in our playroom with and without their siblings present indicate that the presence of a sibling has an effect comparable with that of a peer. In all, then, it may be incorrect to assume that because there is little direct interaction between infants and siblings, siblings play an insignificant role in the infants development. Rather, they appear to facilitate or provide experiences that are unlikely to occur in the course of parent-infant interaction. The most obvious impact is likely to be upon mastery of the object environment.

23

Maternal Employment and Mother-Child Interaction

SARALE E. COHEN

The effects of maternal employment on young children is a frequently debated, yet infrequently studied, issue. Increasing maternal employment makes its effects of great practical as well as theoretical interest. The *Handbook of Labor Statistics* (1976) indicates that the proportion of preschool children whose mothers work has shown a rapid rise, from 18 percent in 1948, to 20 percent in 1960, to 29 percent in 1970, and up to 37 percent in 1976. Recent review articles (Etaugh 1974; Hoffman 1974; Howell 1974; Wallston 1973) have summarized research on maternal employment and indicate that the amount of research in this area with young children has been slight. Etaugh (1974) pointed out that although more concern is expressed as to the effect of maternal employment on young children, more research attention has been directed at the older children.

Few systematic studies of the effects of maternal employment on very young children are available, although data bearing on the issue indirectly are available. Hypotheses may be derived from studies of maternal deprivation, day care, polymatric rearing, and surrogate care-giving. It has been noted that caution is called for, however, in extrapolating from these studies, since institutionalization, day care, and multiple mothering are not the same thing as maternal employment (Hoffman 1974). Many confounding variables are introduced in these kinds of comparisons. It is only very recently that research has been directed at the kinds of interaction that working and nonemployed mothers engage in with their children (Hock 1976). Does the mother-child dyad where the mother has made a regular commitment outside the home behave the same as the mother-child dyad where the mother does not work? In Hock's (1976) study of mothers and children in the first year of life, the employed and nonemployed groups were similar in the behaviors observed. The significance of the issue requires replication as well as an extension of research into the period of early childhood. The present study represents such an extension to the second year of life by describing mother-child interactions that occurred between mothers and their 21-month-old-children in a semi-structured laboratory setting. Additionally, this study examined a prototypic risk group—prematurely born children. The data were obtained as part of a longitudinal study of preterm children; the assessment of maternal employment effects was not part of the original design. The present study has not controlled all the variables that would be desired from a project originally designed to test the employment issue. Its results were derived from a post hoc analysis and warrant consideration.

Method

Subjects

The subjects were part of a longitudinal study of preterm children. The 44 children included in this report met the following criteria: singletons or surviving singletons; free of major neurological, sensory, or motor problems; from English-speaking families; information available to classify mother's employment history. Information regarding maternal employment was obtained primarily from nurses' records which were made during medical checkups that were regularly scheduled for all project children. In addition, supplemental information was available from interviews by a social worker.

The subjects were divided into two groups—mothers employed and mothers not employed. Maternal employment criteria consisted of the following: mother employed or attending school full time at the time of the mother-child interaction observation at 21 months; employment consisted of a minimum of two full days a week or its equivalent; and employment must have been for a duration greater than 8 weeks. About half the working mothers began to work or returned to work before the child was six months old. All but three in the employed group were working by the time the child was one year old. The unemployed mothers were those who were not employed since the birth of the study child. Mothers who did not clearly fit into these two categories were excluded from the present analyses.

There were 14 boys and 8 girls in each group. The two groups did not differ statistically in maternal age, years of maternal education, or in distribution of birth order. The number of families that were single-parent families for some of the child's first 21 months was higher ($N = 7$) for the employed group than for the nonemployed ($N = 1$).

Procedure

The children and their mothers were observed in a laboratory situation when the children were 21 months old. The appointments were scheduled at a time convenient for each mother and child. There was no known bias for employed mothers, as appointments were made on weekends or days off for the employed mothers. The interactional situation consisted of four mother-child interactional tasks which varied in the amount of structuring. The mother and child were seated side by side at a small table, and the mother was instructed to play with and talk to her child as she normally did. The four tasks were as follows: dramatic play, dressing task, book task, and block building. The tasks were presented in an invariant order for a set length of time. Three of the tasks lasted 4 minutes each and the dressing task was of 2 minutes duration. In the dramatic play task a collection of miniature dramatic materials (baby doll, high chair, tub, crib, spoon, dog, and car) were placed on the table and the mother and child were told, "Here are some things for you to play with." The dressing task consisted of a pair of children's mittens being placed on the table and the mother was asked to show the child how to put them on and to try to get the child to do so. The book task consisted of 2 picture books with simple text accompanied by the instructions, "Would you please spend a few minutes looking at books together?" The last interactional task involved two identical sets of blocks and a picture of a simple construction. The mother was asked to show the child how to build the construction and to attempt to get the child to do so. The tester did not participate in the tasks other than to present the materials and instructions.

The interactional tasks were videotaped and were scored from the videotapes. The behaviors observed consisted of 3 major categories: mothers behaviors, child behaviors, and reciprocal interactions involving both members of the dyad. Verbal and nonverbal behaviors were scored. Several behaviors were noted in each category. Those behaviors considered in this report are:

Mother behaviors:

Positive attentiveness to child: any positive verbalization to child such as comment, question, praise, suggest, vocalize contingently, imitate, focus verbally; plus help, facilitate, provide, affectionate touch, positive stance to child's demanding bid.

Negative attentiveness to child: interfering touch, directive prohibition, criticism, ignore or reject child's demanding bid.

Child behaviors:

Vocalization: non-distress vocalization, comprehensible or incomprehensible.

Negative responsiveness: fuss/cry, hit, throw, prohibit, reject mother's bid.

Reciprocal behaviors:

Reciprocal positive attentiveness between mother and child: either member of the dyad responds positively to positive behavior of other (e.g., question and answer, vocalize contingently to other's vocalization, vocalize imitatively, mother's stance positive to child's bid, child complies with mother's suggestion).

The scoring consisted of a combination of time and event sampling. Behaviors of each mother and child dyad were continuously time-sampled in 15 second intervals; consequently, 56 observation intervals were recorded for each dyad. Each behavior was scored as occurring or not within that interval.

Developmental examination. Assessments of competence were made by independent examiners unaware of the mother-child data. The children were tested at 18 months with the Bayley Mental Scale and at 24 months with the Gesell Developmental Schedules. They were also tested with a measure of receptive language and with the Bayley Mental Scale at 25 months.

Results

Laboratory Interaction

In order to compare mother-child behaviors, two-way analyses of variance (Sex X Employment group) were done for selected variables. As table 23.1 indicates, there were differences between the employment groups on each major category. Moth-

Table 23.1 Mean Frequency of Mother-Child Interactional Behaviors

	Employed N = 22	Not Employed N = 22	p
Mother			
positive attentiveness	43.5	48.7	.021
negative attentiveness	17.2	15.1	.210
Child			
vocalization	27.2	36.1	.01
negative responsiveness	10.8	7.8	.148
Reciprocal			
reciprocal positive	23.7	31.2	.002

ers who were not employed gave more positive attentiveness to their children. In turn, the children of the mothers who were not employed vocalized more to their mothers. Additionally, there were more reciprocal social interactions between nonemployed mothers and their children. Differences between the groups were not found in negative behaviors of either the mother or the child. The only sex difference between the groups was in the amount of vocalization—girls vocalized more than boys (girls' $\overline{X} = 36.4$ and boys' $\overline{X} = 28.8$; $F(1,40) = 7.15$, $p < .05$). There were no significant interactions between sex and employment group in mother-child behaviors.

Developmental Examinations

Two way analyses of variance (Employment group X Sex) were done for the assessments of competence. Three of the four developmental tests in the second year of life indicated differences between the employed and not-employed groups. The children whose mothers were not employed scored higher on the Bayley Mental Scale at 18 and 25 months and on the Gesell Development Schedules at 24 months. The two groups did not differ significantly on the measure of receptive language, although, as in the other tests, the not-employed group scored higher. The mean scores are presented in table 23.2. The girls scored significantly higher on the Gesell Developmental Schedules and there were no significant interactions of sex and employment groups.

Table 23.2 Mean Scores on Developmental Tests

	Employed N = 22	Not Employed N = 22	p
Bayley Mental Scale—18 months	90.6	107.3	.000
Gesell—24 months	95.8	106.0	.006
Receptive Language	91.6	104.5	.125
Bayley Mental Scale—25 months	94.6	116.5	.000

Early Measures

The question arises: were these mothers and children different to begin with? No maternal personality data are available. However, a number of observations of the children and of the mothers and children had been made during the first year of life and the two groups were compared.

Analyses of perinatal measures showed a difference between the two groups of children in birth weight. The children of the employed mothers weighed less at birth (mother employed, $\overline{X}$ = 1698 grams; mother not employed, $\overline{X}$ = 2081 grams). In order to determine if the differences between employment groups could be explained by the differences in birth weight, analyses of covariance were done for each of the significant mother-child interaction and competence variables using birth weight as a covariate. Regardless of birth weight, the significant differences remained between the two employment groups. Furthermore, birth weight itself was not significantly correlated with any of the developmental tests nor with the mother-child variables that differentiated the two groups. Thus, birth weight does not appear to be the factor accounting for the group differences in either interaction or competence. Length of hospitalization was also compared and was not significantly different between the two groups. Further, although at 18 months the children of the employed mothers scored significantly lower, analysis of the Gesell Developmental Schedules administered at 9 months indicated no differences between the groups (18 of the 22 employed mothers were working by the time the children were 9 months old). The children of the not-employed group scored 101.8 and the children of the employed group 99.1.

Additionally, measures of the child's social experiences with the mother in the first year were available, as caregiver-child interaction had been observed in the home at 1, 3, and 8 months. Two of the six variables at the 8-month visit were significantly different($p < .05$) according to the univariate *t* tests. The children of the not employed group scored higher than the employed group on face-to-face talks and mutual gazing (mother not employed = .06 and .10, mother employed = .04 and .07 respectively). Thus, in most ways the mothers and children interacted similarly in the first year of life with a difference in reciprocal social interactions beginning to occur at the 8-month visit.

Intactness of Family

Although the mothers of the employed group did not differ in age and years of education from those of the not-employed group, the groups did differ as to the number of parents living in the home throughout the first 21 months of the child's life. The data pertaining to this factor were not systematically collected, however, and the exact duration of the child being reared by one parent cannot be specified. The duration varied from a few weeks to a number of months for several homes. From the information available, the mother's employment usually preceded the breakup of the nuclear family rather than following the father's departure from the home. In order to examine the possibility that the employment effects were due to the single parent aspect of the family, the data were reexamined comparing the 15 "family intact" employed mothers to the 21 "family intact" not-employed mothers. Univariate *t* tests comparing these two groups were done for each of the variables that showed differences between employment groups in the previous analyses. Significant differences were still obtained in the developmental tests and in child vocalization. The children of the not-employed "family intact" mothers scored significantly higher than the children of the employed "family intact" mothers. The developmental test results were as follows with the mean of the not-employed "family intact" presented first in each case: Bayley MDI, 18 months ($\overline{X}$ = 106.5 and $\overline{X}$ = 90.5, $p < .01$); Gesell Developmental Schedules ($\overline{X}$ = 105.5 and $\overline{X}$ = 95.8, $p < .05$); and Bayley MDI, 25 months ($\overline{X}$ = 115.3 and $\overline{X}$ = 96.1, $p < .01$). Additionally, the children of the not-employed "family intact" group emitted more non-distress vocalization at 21 months ($\overline{X}$ = 35.9 and $\overline{X}$ = 27.5, $p < .05$). With respect to the variables maternal positive attentiveness and reciprocal positive interaction, the groups did not show differences as marked as the original comparisons. There was no longer a significant difference in positive attentiveness of the mother (not-employed intact, $\overline{X} = 48.5$, employed intact, $\overline{X} = 44.6$, $p < .10$). However, reciprocal positive attentiveness involving both the mother and the child was of borderline significance with the not-employed intact being higher in this mutual category (not-employed intact, $\overline{X} = 30.7$, employed intact, $\overline{X} = 24.7$, $p < .07$).

Discussion

The results of this study show that dyadic interaction, particularly the child's responsiveness, and developmental status were different for the children of employed and nonemployed mothers in the second year of life. Although a number of measures were found to be significantly related to maternal employment in the total sample, the conclusions must be considered tentative. Caution is necessary in generalizing from these results due to the size and nature of the sample, the post hoc analysis, and the possible confounding of variables with employment status as in the case of birth weight and intactness of family. In comparing only those families that were intact, the employed mothers were no longer significantly different from the unemployed mothers in their positive attentiveness to the child. Single parent families, however, were not an adequate explanation for the differences between the employment groups in behaviors that measured the child's responses such as non-distress vocalization and the child's cognitive functioning in the second year of life. Regardless of the intactness of the family unit, the children of the employed group performed less adequately. To equate for family intactness may result in a loss of important information as to the typical correlates of maternal employment and consequences associated with the actual employment. Approximately one-third of the employed mothers were single parents for part of the first 21 months. Thus, single-parent families seem to reflect a reality of the maternal employment situation with very young children.

A typical concern has been with the care that the child of the working mother receives during the mother's absence. The nature of the substitute care is of paramount importance. This study suggests that it is also important that we examine the nature of the maternal care itself, the interchanges that occur between working mothers and their young children, and the child's social and cognitive development. This is not to suggest that all children of working mothers are adversely affected. Nevertheless, this descriptive study raises some questions about the effects of maternal employment during the child's first two years. These questions deal not only with the effect on the child's cognitive functioning and social responses, but also with a potential effect on the mother's behavior to the child. In the laboratory interaction, it is somewhat artificial to separate the mother's behavior from the child's since they are an interactive system; however, the data suggest that the employed mother may be eliciting or receiving fewer responses from her child.

The premature children in this study present a group that is considered at risk for developmental problems (Drillien 1964). It is possible that the effects of maternal employment may be heightened in such vulnerable groups. On the other hand, it may be that the second year of life is a sensitive period in which the effects of employment on the child may be particularly pronounced. The questions raised by this study merit systematic investigation and suggest that further study of maternal employment is necessary. It would be desirable to study maternal employment effects in the early childhood period in normal populations as well as in groups considered at risk for biological and social factors.

24

The Effects of Day Care

A Critical Review

JAY BELSKY AND LAURENCE D. STEINBERG

Increasing rates of single parenthood and maternal employment in recent decades have sparked concomitant increases in the need for and utilization of alternative care arrangements for children (*Child Care Data and Materials* 1974). Not surprisingly, these changes have themselves generated a great deal of concern in the minds of policymakers, program administrators, human developmentalists, and parents about the short- and long-term consequences of day care. Our purpose here is to review critically the evidence amassed to date on this issue. We have, so to speak, some good news and some bad: the good news is that the number of investigations examining the effects of alternative care arrangements has increased substantially during the past 8 years; the bad news is that, when considered from a broader perspective on human development, we know shockingly little about the impact of day care on children, on their parents, and on the society in which these children and parents live.

Part of this ignorance is due to a near-exclusive reliance on standardized tests of intellectual and social development whose usefulness in understanding development in real-life settings has been repeatedly questioned, most recently by Bronfenbrenner

(1977), Ginsburg and Koslowski (1976), and McCall (1977). Part is due to inherent limitations in evidence derived from studies of only high-quality, university-based day care,which is atypical of the alternative care arrangements utilized by most parents. But, primarily, our ignorance is due to a persistent and pervasive narrowness of scope in day-care reseach that has virtually limited studies of the consequences of day care to investigations of the direct effects of the day-care experience on the individual child. Rarely are the effects of day care on parents and on other social institutions examined, although common sense tells us that such consequences must exist and must also be profound, not only for parents and institutions but for children as well.

The review that follows is organized around the domains of outcomes most often investigated in studies of the effects of day care: the cognitive, emotional, and social development of the child.

Major Findings

Cogntive Development

The effects of day care upon the intellectual development of the child have been extensively researched, but almost exclusively with children enrolled in well-funded, high-quality, university-based programs, often conducted with the specific goal of providing "cognitive enrichment" for their enrollees. (One notable exception to this is the *New York City Infant Day Care Study* [Golden et al. 1978]). Data derived from such programs must therefore be interpreted with certain qualifications in mind. The overall picture of evidence, duly qualified, suggests that the day-care experience has neither salutary nor adverse effects on the intellectual development (as measured by standardized tests) of most children. For economically disadvantaged children, however, day care may have an enduring positive effect, for it appears that such day-care experience may attenuate the declines in test scores typically associated with high-risk populations after 18 months of age (Golden & Birns 1976).

Effects on low-risk children. An overwhelming majority of studies of the effects of day care on subsequent intellectual development have indicated no differences between day-care-reared children and matched controls (Caldwell et al. 1970; Cochran 1977; Moore 1975; Doyle & Somers 1977; Kagan, Kearsley, and Zelazo 1976; Fowler & Khan 1974; Saunders 1972; Lewis 1975; Prentice & Bieri 1970). Although a number of these investigators had found initial gains in one or many test subscales (e.g., Fowler & Kahn 1975), all significant differences between day-care children and matched controls disappeared during the program or soon after termination. For children from relatively advantaged families, then, exposure to day care, even to high-quality, cognitively enriched programs, does not appear to result in any long-term gains in test performance. We emphasize, however, that neither does it seem that any losses in intellectual performance result from enrollment in day care.

Advantages for disadvantaged children. Significant positive effects of the day-care experience on performance on standardized tests of intellectual development have been reported by a handful of investigators for those children who have been categorized as higher risk than the average middle-class child. It should be noted, however, that most of the programs in which these children were enrolled were specifically designed to provide cognitive enrichment, although they varied widely in the type and degree of special enrichment provided for the children and families involved (see Heber et al. 1972; Robinson & Robinson 1971). Lally (1973; 1974), for example, found that day-care children from poorly educated families performed better on the Stanford-Binet given under optimal conditions than did their matched home-reared counterparts, but that controls from well-educated families scored even higher than the matched day-care group. More importantly, while 29 percent of the low-education, home-reared group obtained an IQ below 90 on the test, only 7 percent of the day-care group did so; none of the high-education controls scored in this range. On the basis of these results, it would appear that an enriching day-care experience may attenuate some of the adverse effects typically associated with high-risk environments.

Further support for this conclusion is provided in a series of reports by Ramey and his colleagues (Ramey & Smith 1976; Ramey & Mills 1975) emanating from their longitudinal study of three groups of infants: (1) a high-risk experimental group enrolled in a specially designed cognitive enrichment day-care program; (2) a high-risk, home-reared control group matched to the experimentals on a number of important variables (e.g., social class, age, sex, race), and (3) a general population contrast group reared at home in more economically advantaged families. During the period when the infants were between 6 and 18 months old, performance on the mental developmental subscale of the Bayley Infant Test declined for the high-risk controls (from 104 to 86), while it remained stable (near 104) for the high-risk experimentals (Ramey & Smith 1976). In addition, motor development subscale scores on this same test revealed significant differences between these two groups favoring the day-care-reared children. Moreover, the scores of these experimental children were not significantly different from those of children in the economically more advantaged, general population contrast group.

In the follow-up investigation, Ramey and Campbell (1977) demonstrated that these patterns of decline in the level of functioning for the home-reared, economically disadvantaged children and stability for their day-care-reared counterparts continue into the children's third year. They reported that the high-risk controls' mean Binet score dropped to 83 at 24 months and 81 at 36 months, while their day-care counterparts' mean remained between 90 and 100 during this same time period (94 at 24 months; 96 at 36 months). As noted earlier, it does not seem to be the case that the IQ scores of high-risk children enrolled in day care increase as a function of their day-care experience; rather, the evidence indicates that a specially designed day-care experience may lessen the decline in IQ typically found for children from economically disadvantaged populations.

Effects of different forms of care. The recently completed *New York City Infant Day Care Study* (Golden et al. 1978) provides evidence which suggests that the benefits accruing to high-risk children from day-care experience may not be restricted to those enrolled in high-quality, cognitively enriched, university-sponsored programs. Analyses of the scores on the Bayley Mental Development Index (MDI) (at 18 months), Stanford-Binet (at 36 months), and Peabody Picture Vocabulary Test (also at 36 months) of approximately 400 children reared at home or enrolled in one of the 31 service-oriented, licensed, public and private, community-controlled, group and family infant day-care programs in New York City reveal consistent differences between children as a function of rearing experience.

At 18 months, children who had been enrolled in child care outside the home between the ages of 2 and 14 months outperformed their home-reared counterparts on the Bayley MDI ($\bar{X}$s = 100.4, 98.0, 92.9, for center day care, family day care, and home day care, respectively). While only the differences between the center- and home-reared groups were statistically significant at this age ($p < .01$), by 36 months, the performance of center-reared children ($\bar{X} = 99.1$) on the Stanford-Binet differed significantly from both family day-care-reared ($\bar{X} = 92.0$) and home-reared children ($\bar{X} = 92.6$). Since the maximum difference between groups is only 7 points and therefore of questionable functional significance, caution is required in interpreting these findings. Nevertheless, the results emerging from this investigation of modal day care in New York City do indicate, consistent with the findings of Ramey and his collaborators, that experience in group day care may prevent the decline in intellectual performance (as assessed by standard IQ tests) generally manifested by low-income children after 18 months of age. The importance of the *New York City Infant Day Care Study* is that it provides evidence about the possible intellectual benefits of day care for infants from high-risk populations who are enrolled in modal (rather than model) care programs.

In sum, existing evidence warrants the conclusion that, so far as intelligence as measured by standardized tests is concerned, experience in day-care programs meeting present federal and state standards has little positive or negative effect on children from advantaged families. Center-based programs which serve high-risk children do, however, appear to succeed in attenuating the declines in test scores typically associated with these disadvantaged populations. We have virtually no information regarding variations in the type or quality of the day care experience and how these variations may affect intellectual development and little evidence on how day care affects intelligence which is not measured by standardized tests. There is an urgent need to assess the impact of day care on functional intelligence in real-life settings.

Emotional Development

Historically, the mother-child bond has been a prime focus of concern to those interested in the influence of early experience upon emotional development. Psychoanalytic theory and prior research on institutionalized children (e.g., Baer 1954; Bowlby 1951; Goldfarb 1943; Spitz 1945) has suggested that any arrangement that deprives the child of continuous access to the mother impairs the development of a strong maternal attachment and thereby adversely affects the child's emotional security. Since day care, by its very nature, entails the daily separation of mother from child, a good deal of attention has been devoted to discovering whether child care outside the home does disrupt the child's emotional tie to his or her mother.

In investigating this important issue, researchers have primarily relied upon some variant of Ainsworth and Wittig's (1969) "strange-situation" experiment, in which a stressful situation is created by repeatedly separating the child from his mother and/or introducing him to a strange adult. The assumption is that the child's approach-avoidance responses to his mother and to the stranger, as well as his exploration of the environment, index the quality of the mother-child relationship.

In this review of studies examining the impact of day care upon emotional development, we first consider investigations employing the strange-situation experiment that have found reliable differences in attachment behavior between children reared in day care versus at home. Next, we shall review those researches that have employed this same methodology, but have failed to discern reliable day-care/home-care differences. Finally, before drawing any conclusions regarding the impact of day care on the mother-child bond, we shall discuss other research using somewhat different methodologies to examine the relationship between type of care and the mother-child bond.

Attachment to mother as a function of type of care. Blehar (1974), in a study of 40 children between 2 and 4 years of age from intact, middle-class families reported the first and only data purporting to show that day care may adversely affect the child's relationship with his mother. Half of her sample had been enrolled for approximately 5 months in private day-care centers. The remainder were reared at home. When compared in the strange situation, the 40-month-old day-care children manifested "anxious-ambivalent" attachments to their mothers (less exploration prior to separation, more crying and more searching during separation, and more proximity seeking and resistance behavior to mother upon reunion), while 30-month-olds manifested "anxious-avoidant" attachments (more resistance and avoidance behavior and less proximity seeking during reunion).

In a recent attempt to replicate Blehar's results, Moskowitz, Schwarz, and Corsini (1977) studied a group of 42-month-olds who had averaged 5 months in day care and a group of matched home-reared controls. In marked contrast to Blehar's findings, these researchers found that the home-reared children rather than the day-care children exhibited more distress upon separation from mother. Moreover, the two groups were indistinguishable in the behavior displayed toward mother prior to and after separation.

Two researchers (Cochran 1977; Ricciuti 1974, study B) working with children 1 year of age, have, like Blehar and unlike Moskowitz, Schwarz, and Corsini, reported greater distress reactions for day-care-reared than home-reared children during separation from the mother. In a study of children enrolled in an experimental nursery at Cornell University, Ricciuti attributed an observed difference in crying to a methodological artifact. Instead of being dropped off by mother in the day-care nursery as was the usual practice, for purposes of the experiment the day-care children were left by their mothers in a strange room. In Ricciuti's view, the excess crying of the day-care sample was more likely a function of this incongruous experience than any disturbance in the children's attachment to their mothers.

In Cochran's (1977) Swedish study, separation procedures were conducted in the home rather than in the laboratory. In discussing his results, Cochran makes the important point that the similarities in behavior between groups far outweighed the observed differences in response to the strange situation. In her small sample study, Ragozin (1977) makes a similar point in noting that only 2 of 14 measures from the strange situation differentiated between home-reared and day-care-reared 1½–3-year olds.

In contrast to the results of the Ricciuti and Cochran investigations, an unpublished study by Doyle and Somers (1977) presents data indicating that home-reared infants cried more and played less during separation from mother than did their day-care-reared counterparts. Two points should be noted in considering the findings of this investigation. First, infants in this research averaged 22 months of age rather than 12 as in the Ricciuti and Cochran investigations. More important, the home-reared and day-care-reared samples were not as carefully matched in this experiment as in the other studies mentioned.

In summary, the research purporting to show home-care/day-care differences in the children's attachments to their mothers is contradictory. Blehar's (1974), Ricciuti's (1974), and Cochran's (1977) data can be interpreted as evidence in favor of home-reared children; the Moskowitz, Schwarz, and Corsini (1977) and Doyle and Somers (1977) data, in contrast, show differences in favor of day-care-reared children.

In addition to studies discerning differences between home-reared and day-care-reared children in the strange situation, there are a number of investigations, often using this same methodology, that have yielded negative findings (i.e., no rearing-group differences).

In the very first study aimed at examining the impact of day care on the child's relation with his mother, Caldwell et al. (1970) evaluated the attachment relationship in a sample of 41 2½-year-olds, 18 of whom had been enrolled in a high-quality, university-affiliated center from the time they were about 1 year old. Most of the subjects were from lower-class families. The assessment consisted of child-mother attachment ratings on seven scales (e.g., dependency, hostility, nurturance, affiliation) made by a staff member after an intensive, semistructured interview with the mother in which the child was present. When ratings for the day-care sample were compared with those for 22 home-reared control children, no significant group differences were discerned.

Four recent investigations employing the strange situation, one of 10–12-month-olds (Brookhart & Hock 1976), another of 5–30-month-olds (Doyle 1975), a third of 36-month-olds (Roopnarine & Lamb 1978), and a fourth of 41–45-month-olds (Portnoy & Simmons 1978), have also failed to discern day-care/home-care differences.

The Portnoy and Simmons (1978) attempt to replicate Blehar's findings and examine the effects of age of entry into day care is of special interest. In finding no rearing-group differences between (1) children reared entirely at home (equivalent to Blehar's home-reared sample), (2) children reared until 3 years at home and then enrolled in center day care (equivalent to Blehar's day care sample), and (3) children reared at home until 1, placed in family day care until 3, and then transferred to center day care (a group included to test age-of-entry effects), these investigators concluded that not only does age of entry into day care not systematically affect children's attachments to their mothers, but also that Blehar's findings may have been an artifact of "a transient distress reaction associated with new day care arrangement" (p. 241). Since the children in their study averaged 5 months of additional day-care experience before being tested in the strange situation relative to Blehar's sample (9.45 vs. 4.78), Portnoy and Simmons concluded that their failure to replicate Blehar's findings casts doubt on the notion that there are long-range effects of day care on the mother-child attachment relationship.

In the most comprehensive and best controlled study to date, Kagan, Kearsley, and Zelazo (1976) compared 32 pairs of children matched for sex, ethnicity (Caucasian-Chinese), and social class (working-middle), half of whom were enrolled in full-time care between the ages of 3½ and 30 months. Again, the day-care children in this study, like those in the Caldwell et al. (1970) and Ricciuti (1974) researches, were cared for in a university-sponsored, research-oriented center, thus assuring a high caregiver-child ratio and high-quality care. Periodic assessments made between the ages of 3½ and 29 months indicated that children reared in home versus day care did not differ in crying behavior when separated from the mother in a laboratory situation.

The caretaker-child relationship. In a number of investigations, an alternative approach has been taken to examine the impact of day care on the child's emotional development. These alternative methods address rather different questions than those posed by investigators using the strange situation, namely: (1) Does the day-care child develop an attachment-like relationship with his caregiver? and (2) Does the day-care child become more attached to his caregiver than to his mother? Procedures aimed at finding answers to these questions have focused upon determining the child's preference for his mother, his caregiver, or a strange adult.

In a longitudinal study of children enrolled in the Cornell Experimental Nursery, Ricciuti (1974, study A) explored both questions posed above. Monthly examinations of infants' responses to being left by their mother in the presence of a strange adult and/or a familiar caregiver provided evidence that infants can develop a discriminating attachment-like relationship toward the latter. However, this relationship did not replace or supersede the child's emotional bond with his mother.

Working with a sample of poor, black children, age 9–31 months (albeit enrolled in a high-quality, university-sponsored center), Farran and Ramey (1977), using a different methodology than Ricciuti's, drew conclusions somewhat similar to his. Behavior recordings made when the day-care children were placed in a laboratory setting with mother, caregiver, and strange adult indicated that the children were more likely to interact with their mothers (e.g., offering toys, touching) than with their caregiver. Moreover, when confronted with the problem-solving task of obtaining a cookie from a tightly sealed container, all 15 of the

23 children who requested help turned to their mothers for such assistance.

The Kagan, Kearsley, and Zelazo (1976) study employed a somewhat similar procedure for comparing the adult preferences of day-care-reared and home-reared children. Boredom and stress were built into a laboratory situation by providing few toys with which the child could play and by directing the three adults in the room to switch seats twice during a 15-minute observation period. Once again, findings indicated that children, home-reared and day-care-reared alike, expressed strong preferences for their mothers.

In sum, the total body of evidence reviewed regarding the effect of day care on the child's attachment to his mother offers little support for the claim that day care disrupts the child's tie to his mother. With the exception of Blehar's (1974) report, not a single study provided evidence documenting the existence of substantial, systematic differences between day-care-reared and home-reared children in behavior displayed in the strange situation or in some modified version of this procedure. And, given Moskowitz, Schwarz, and Corsini's (1977) and Portnoy and Simmons's (1978) failure to replicate Blehar's findings once rigorous experimental controls were included in the study design, one can only be left to question the validity, let alone the generalizability, of this single exception to the general trend.

The absence of evidence for deleterious effects of day care in existing research does not mean, however, that no such effects occur. It is important to remember that most investigations reviewed (Caldwell et al. 1970; Farran & Ramey 1977; Ricciuti 1974; Kagan, Kearsley, and Zelazo 1976) involved children from day-care programs which may not be representative of those available to most parents, namely, centers run by universities for research purposes and providing high-quality care. Given the prevalence of studies involving superior environments, effects of modal day care in America on the mother-child bond remain unknown. Nevertheless, we can conclude from the research reviewed that, given high-quality day care, significant disruption of the mother-child bond (as measured by the strange situation) does not appear likely. Nor is there any reason to conclude that the enrollment of infants in high-quality day care leads to the replacement of the mother by the caregiver as the child's primary object of attachment.

Social Development

When a group of Massachusetts parents were asked to indicate their most important concerns regarding outcomes of substitute care, they most often replied that the program should help their children get along with others, a value which may be distinctive for American socialization (Bronfenbrenner 1970). In keeping with this emphasis, research on the social outcomes of day care focuses primarily on the relation of the child with his peers.

Relations with peers. In general, studies of the peer relations of day-care and non-day-care children indicate that at early and later ages there may be a tendency for day-care children to be more peer oriented, although a few investigators have not found this difference. In one set of studies, children were individually placed in a play situation with their mothers and one or more unfamiliar age-mates. The focus of attention was the extent to which each child was willing to leave the mother and initiate interaction with other children. In an experiment by Ricciuti (1974, study D), day-care infants (12–19 months) exceeded matched home-reared controls in the distance moved away from mother during the first 2 minutes of observation and in the distance they maintained throughout the experimental period. Moreover, the day-care children were more visually oriented toward the other children and less so toward their mothers, and engaged in less sustained physical contact with their mothers than their home-reared counterparts. Ratings of general affective state (positive, negative, or neutral), however, revealed no differences between home-care and day-care infants, as both groups remained close to neutral.

Kagan, Kearsley, and Zelazo (1976) found that when mothers returned to a playroom in which their children were playing with a peer, home-reared 20-month-olds show a greater increase in their proximity to their mothers than did their day-care counterparts. These same authors report similar but nonsignificant trends at 29 months. Employing a procedure similar to that used by Ricciuti (1974, study D), these investigators found that home-reared children were more apprehensive (played less with toys) than their day-care counterparts, though they did not differ from them in proximity and visual orientation as Ricciuti reported. This discrepancy may be due to the fact that the children in the Kagan investigation were 4–8 months older than those studied by Ricciuti, and visual orientation may not have been as important an indication of peer attraction for these older children.

Summary

As we have suggested earlier, although research on day care has increased substantially in volume in the last 8 years, it has remained surprisingly narrow in scope. In consequence, the results of this review can be summarized in relatively brief compass. With regard to children's intellectual development, the available evidence indicates, in general, that day care has neither beneficial nor deleterious effects. For children growing up in high-risk environments, however, experience in center-based care does appear to attenuate the declines in IQ frequently observed in youngsters from economically disadvantaged backgrounds. With regard to emotional development, the weight of the evidence indicates that day care is not disruptive of the child's emotional bond with his mother, even when day care is initiated in the first year of life. In addition, there is no indication that exposure to day care decreases the child's preference for his mother in comparison with an alternative familiar caregiver. Finally, with respect to social development, the existing data indicate that day-care-reared children, when compared with agemates reared at home, interact more with peers in both positive and negative ways.

PART VI

Early Intervention

Much of the scientific study of infancy, and indeed many of the papers included in this volume, highlight environmental forces and transactional processes that influence the quality of early human development. Serious consideration of this work suggests a variety of strategies for intervening to enhance early development. In this final section, two approaches for early intervention are detailed. Ramey and Campbell describe a center-based program that provides full-day care to infants from economically impoverished homes. The program, which offers a highly structured and carefully planned curriculum for fostering both cognitive and social development, has been in existence for almost 10 years. Since the children are enrolled in the program early in their first year and remain in the center until they reach school age, Ramey and his colleagues have been able to carefully chart the children's development for purposes of determining the effects of the program. The results of this evaluation, through the children's fourth birthdays, are summarized in the selection printed here. As the reader will no doubt recognize, the program has been successful, as the children enrolled in it are performing at levels far superior to those of a group of matched controls cared for in their own impoverished homes.

The second paper in this section describes a radically different, but no less comprehensive, approach to early intervention. Like Ramey's center-based program, David Olds' Prenatal/Early Infancy Project represents an effort to prevent developmental disabilities. Starting early in pregnancy, Olds' program provides home-visiting services by nurses to women at risk for childbearing and childrearing difficulties. This support continues after the child is born and through the second year of life. The specific function of the home-visiting service changes as both mother and child grow in order to provide support and guidance that is appropriate to the developmental tasks that both mother and child face.

In addition to working directly with the mother, the home visitor is trained to work with other members of the child's immediate and extended family, and with those formal and informal social supports (e.g., Childbirth Education Association, local church, mother's peer group) that can also be of assistance to her. The fact that Olds' program directs its energies not only at the mother and child, but to the context in which they are embedded as well, leads Olds to appropriately describe his project as an ecological intervention.

Unlike Ramey's program, which has generated much evaluation data, Olds' program is relatively new and evaluation of it is in an early stage. As Olds indicates, however, the research program attached to this service is so well conceptualized that it will not only be possible to determine whether the intervention positively influences children and their families, but also to identify the social and psychological processes by which the program exerts its effects. Such knowledge, it should be pointed out, is essential if Olds' work is to be of assistance to efforts to streamline his and other programs so as to ensure maximum effectiveness at minimum costs.

25

Compensatory Education for Disadvantaged Children

CRAIG T. RAMEY AND
FRANCES A. CAMPBELL

Poverty is expensive. Moreover, the costs of poverty go far beyond the immediate loss of revenues to the state. They extend into the futures of parents and their children. An all too frequent consequence of economic deprivation and the accompanying alienation from the mainstream of American life is an intellectual and social deficit that perpetuates itself from generation to generation. A self-perpetuating and downward social spiral is set up in some families such that the consequences of extreme poverty in one generation create a set of circumstances which prevent parents from adequately ministering to their children's social and intellectual needs. This lack of social nurturance results in delayed development which puts the child at a serious disadvantage compared with his more affluent classmates upon entry into public school. The initial disadvantage and the family's continuing isolation from the community's cultural and social mainstream create a poor prognosis for the child's educational and social future.

In recognition of the cyclic nature of poverty in this country, major national programs for preschool compensatory education were developed in the 1960s. These programs were designed to counter the adverse effects of poverty on young children before they entered the public school system. The basic goal of the early intervention efforts was to ensure that developing children from poverty-level backgrounds received the necessary preschool experiences to allow them to take full advantage of educational opportunities available in public schools. It was hoped that this head start in the educational process would permit them to be academically more competitive.

Recent reviews of early intervention programs (e.g., Bronfenbrenner 1975; Karnes & Teska 1975; Haskins, Finkelstein & Stedman 1978) have presented arguments for early intervention efforts which can be summarized briefly around the following five issues.

1. Can preschool intervention programs result in accelerated developmental growth? Almost without exception, disadvantaged children have shown substantial gains in IQ and other cognitive measures during the first year they were enrolled in a program, frequently attaining or exceeding the average mental growth for children their age (Bronfenbrenner 1975). There does not, however, exist in the scientific literature direct evidence to show that predicted declines in intellectual performance can be prevented during the preschool period for children whose background of poverty places them at high risk for socioculturally caused mental retardation.

2. Can children maintain the rate of intellectual growth when the program ends or the children enter school? It appears that the major gains children make through early education come during the first year of intervention. In subsequent years the youngsters may be able to sustain their new level of ability, but they will often lose the temporary gain unless the stimulating program is continued (Karnes & Teska 1975).

3. What impact did special programs have on social behavior and motivation? Domains other than cognitive performance of children have received scant attention by researchers. Relatively little is known about the effects of early intervention on such important topics as personal-social adjustment, motivation, ability to interact with others, attention to task, and approaches to tasks.

4. Does the nature of the program make a difference? In aggregate, early intervention programs produce intellectual gains, but no one program or group of programs seems to be consistently superior to others (Mann, Harrell, & Hunt 1976). However, cognitively structured curricula produce greater gains than play-oriented nursery schools, according to the review by Bronfenbrenner (1975). Thus more structured programs with specific instructional objectives and strategies to meet those objectives have produced larger positive changes in children.

5. What variables are associated with intellectual gains? Reviews such as Bronfenbrenner's (1975) and Karnes and Teska's (1975) are in agreement that the earlier the instructional program begins in the child's life the better the result. In addition, the more parents participate in the project the more enduring the intellectual gains appear to be. However, the lower the socioeconomic status of the parents the more difficult it is to get and sustain parent participation. This difficulty may account, in part, for the observation that the children who profited least from the programs and showed the most rapid decline were those who came from the most deprived social and economic backgrounds.

The Carolina Abecedarian Project

Conclusions consonant with the reviewers just cited, led, in 1972, to the creation of a multidisciplinary project which was designed to extend our scientific and educational understanding of the factors affecting the growth and development of children from the country's lowest socioeconomic strata. That effort produced a longitudinal, early, and continuing educational program known as the Carolina Abecedarian Project. The Latinate word, Abecedarian, which means one who learns the rudiments of something, was chosen to reflect the basic philosophy undergirding the project's efforts.

The hypotheses underlying this intervention program may be stated as follows: (1) Young children who spend significant amounts of their waking hours in a stable, predictable, and intellectually stimulating environment will develop enhanced competencey in language. This increased competency will concretize their social and physical environment. Mastery of a symbol system will allow children to deal more effectively with complex concepts as the children mature. It follows that such children will show enhanced performance on standardized intellectual tests relative to children not receiving intervention. (2) The intervention program will aid in establishing social communication and confidence.

Operational features. The intervention in the Abecedarian Project consists of an infant and early childhood educational program delivered in a day-care setting where a special curriculum is systematically used to stimulate the children's cognitive and social development.

The Children and Their Families

Families were referred to the project through local hospitals, clinics, and the County Department of Social Services. Once a family had been identified as potentially eligible, the supervisor of the infant nursery visited the home to explain the program and to begin to determine whether the family did, in fact, meet the selection criteria.

The criterion for inclusion consisted of the total score obtained on a high-risk index (Ramey & Smith 1976). That index included such factors as parental education, income, maternal IQ score, history of social or emotional problems, evidence of educational retardation in other family members, intactness of the family, and need for public assistance. These factors were assigned a priori weights based upon their estimated importance. A total score above a certain cutoff point was required for inclusion in the sample.

A crucial feature of the Carolina Abecedarian Project is that the high-risk families were randomly assigned either to the experimental group (those receiving day care at the Frank Porter Graham Center) or to the control group (those who did not receive day care). This was done by matching pairs of mothers on maternal age, IQ, education, and parity, then assigning them randomly to either the experimental or control group.

At the present time, four yearly cohorts of approximately 28 biologically normal children have been admitted to the program. Two, or approximately 2 percent of the sample, are white children; the rest are black. The oldest children in the program are presently 5 years of age and entered kindergarten in the fall of 1977. To date, the population has been quite stable, and parental cooperation with the program has been very good.

Components of the Program

The main difference between the two high-risk groups is that the experimental group receives a planned curriculum administered throughout the day in a day-care setting. Infants in the day-care program begin attending the center as young as 6 weeks of age: attendance must begin by age 3 months. The center operates from 7:45 A.M. to 5:30 P.M. each weekday for 50 weeks per year. A van and two station wagons equipped with child safety seats are used to transport infants and children to and from the center.

Families in both groups receive services designed to reduce the potentially differential effects of extraeducational poverty experiences upon the children's development. These include, for both groups, family-support social work services provided on a need basis at the family's request, nutritional supplements either through the two meals per day routinely given to experimental children at the center or through the provision of free bottled formula for infants up to 15 months of age in the control group, free medical care for all experimental children at the center and for control children at the local primary care clinics and comprehensive health centers, and transportation to and from the center for parents and children taking part in research and evaluation procedures.

Families in both groups are paid for participation in research and evaluation studies. As an incentive for continued participation by the control group, disposable diapers are made available free to these families for up to 3 years. After children are out of diapers, the payment for participation is somewhat larger for control families than for experimental families.

Beginning at age 3 months, both the experimental and control subjects take part in a comprehensive assessment program in which the children are evaluated by the Bayley Scales of Infant Development every 3 months up to age 18 months and standardized intelligence tests every 6 months from age 24 to age 60 months.

Children are evaluated by the Stanford-Binet Intelligence Scale (Terman and Merrill 1973) at 24, 36, and 48 months; the McCarthy Scales of Children's Abilities at 30, 42, and 54 months; and the Wechsler Preschool and Primary Scale of Intelligence at 60 months.

Settings

The center houses children on three floors of a multipurpose building. Prewalking infants are cared for in a suite of four connected rooms on the fourth floor—two are for sleeping and two for play and curriculum activities. The 14 infants typically in this setting are cared for by a head teacher, three assistant teachers, and the nursery supervisor, who is also the person responsible for the initial recruitment of families and maintenance of parent contacts. All teachers care for all infants on an individual need basis. Curriculum assignments for three or four children are given to individual teachers at two-week intervals. Infants pace themselves through the day according to their own eating, sleeping, and waking times.

When infants are able to walk alone with good control, they are gradually moved into the toddler group on the second floor. This transition is accomplished by having a teacher from the infant group accompany the new toddlers as they gradually increase the period of time each day in the toddler group. The teacher fades out her involvement with the transition children by paying more and more attention to others in the group until the new toddlers are fully acclimated to the setting. Children usually graduate to the toddler setting in groups of three or four.

The toddlers' setting is one of four different classrooms housed on the second floor of the building. The classrooms contain four groups of children: the toddlers, two multiage groups, and the 3-year-old group. The different classrooms are divided from one another by large, moveable fiberglass partitions which form low barriers. One side of this floor opens onto a play yard where sandboxes and wheeled toys are available. Inside the building there is also a large common space where climbing and sliding equipment is available. A conference area for teachers is in one corner of this space.

At approximately 2 years of age, when the toddlers have developed more language, they are moved into one of the two multiage groups. The groups are defined as "multiage" because they contain the most verbal of the toddlers, all the 2-year-olds, and older children who, for various reasons, seem unready to move to the 3-year-old class. These groups consist of about eight children with a head teacher and an assistant teacher in each. The play equipment and space arrangements reflect the need for make-believe play, small-group teacher-directed activities, self-directed play and one-to-one interactions with teachers.

The final classroom area on the second floor is designated for 3-year-olds. Eight 3-year-olds and two teachers make up this group. Ten 4-year-olds and their teachers are housed on the first floor of the building in an area which opens onto a large playground. For both 3- and 4-year-olds the classroom space is divided into more formal learning centers devoted to dramatic play, reading, art, music, nature, and science. Each classroom has areas for being alone or playing in small groups. Structured and nonstructured activities are interspersed throughout the day.

Curriculum

The curriculum is designed to provide unambiguous experiences and activities presented in such a way that the children can master them. They foster development in language, motor, social, and cognitive areas. Much of the teaching at all ages occurs in one to one interaction between teacher and child. Individual prescriptions of items are written for each child and revised every two to three weeks.

To provide each child with the prescription best suited to his current needs, teachers keep developmental charts for each child. Once the teacher has determined a given child's status in an area such as language, the teacher searches the curriculum banks for the best match between child status and items. In the Abecedarian program, a curriculum developer assists in this observer/search/match process. After two weeks, during which the chosen items are applied as an integral part of the child's daily routine, new items are chosen or the old ones continued based on the child's progress. Because this procedure is individualized, it helps to document the variety and quantity of each child's actual curriculum experience. This program is formally applied up to a child's third birthday.

When children reach 3 years of age they move into an educational program which draws on a variety of curriculum materials available for preschool education. Resources such as the *Peabody Early Education Kit* (Dunn et al. 1976), *Bridges to Reading* (Greenberg and Epstein 1973), and *GOAL Math Program* (Karnes 1973) are used in skill groups to meet individual children's developmental needs. The teaching staff plans the program, organizes the environment, and guides the use of the material.

Results from the Abecedarian Program

Intellectual Consequences

A major goal of the Abecedarian Project has been to prevent a decline in intellectual development in the experimental group of high-risk children. To date, we have complete longitudinal test data to age 36 months on 54 children and test data at 48 months on the oldest 28 (cohort 1). Recall that the Bayley Scales of Infant Development (1969) were given to the children as infants; the Stanford-Binet Intelligence Scale (Terman and Merrill 1973) has been used annually from 24 months through 48 months of age.

No group differences in Bayley Mental Development Index (MDI) scores have been found up to age 12 months. The control group mean showed a sharp drop on the 18-month MDI score, while the experimental group did not change. These findings have been presented in greater detail by Ramey and Campbell (1977).

A major question posed in the present analysis was whether there was a significant difference in the degree of change shown in the two groups of high-risk children from infancy to preschool age. The means for the two groups are presented in figure 25.1. The mean scores were lower at 36 months than at 12 months in both groups. It is difficult to interpret the meaning of these linear contrasts since the finding is confounded by having not only a

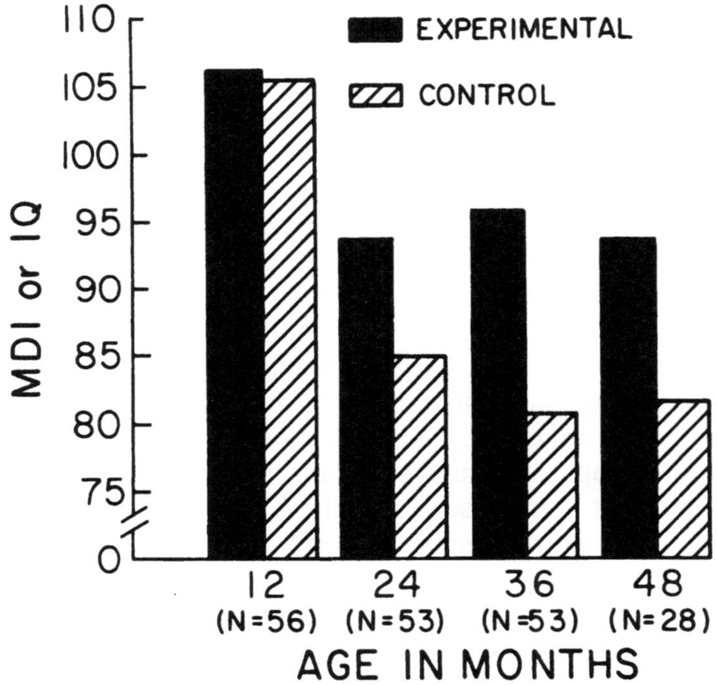

Figure 25.1 Degree of change in two groups of high risk children.

change in age but also a change in the standardized test used at the 12- and the 24- and 36-month test occasions. It is impossible to know, then, whether the decline seen is a real change in intellectual ability over the years from 12 to 36 months or is an artifact of the different tests used.

What is clear, however, is that the two groups changed differently over time. The control group declined significantly more than did the experimental group. There are no group differences at 12 months and significant group differences at each age thereafter.

We examined the individual Binet items to see whether the two groups of children showed differential passing rates on particular classes of items. Disadvantaged children begin to show deficits on tests at the age when spoken language is starting to develop and at the age when tests begin to require more language competence. We hypothesized, therefore, that children in the intervention program would have a language advantage which would help to account for their superior test performance.

Social Consequences

The social consequences of early, supplemental education have also been studied within the Abecedarian Project. We have been primarily concerned about the direct effects of early intervention upon the children's social and emotional development. One of the ways we have studied the developing social behavior of infants has been by rating their behavior in standardized testing situations on the 28 items of the Bayley Infant Behavior Record (IBR). Although a testing situation constitutes a limited sample of infant behavior, it provides one means of making direct comparisons of behaviors exhibited by children of both groups in a standard context.

The IBR items for 79 children assessed at ages 6, 12, and 18 months were subjected to separate principal components factor analyses with varimax rotation to orthogonal structure. Items were defined as loading on a particular factor when loadings were .40 or greater. Two similar factors were obtained at all four ages. These were a unipolar factor measuring goal-directed behavior, persistence, and responsiveness to objects, and a bipolar factor with responsiveness to the examiner and happiness at one pole and fearfulness at the other. These factors were labeled goal-directed behavior and social confidence, respectively.

Factor scores were derived for each child on the two factors described above, and *t*-tests of group means on these were computed. At 6, 12, and 18 months the center-attending children were rated as significantly more socially confident than control children. At 18 months, center-attending children were rated as showing more goal-directed behavior than control children.

These results show that early supplemental education has important benefits for disadvantaged children. We have seen significant declines in tested intellectual development in our nontreated control children, whereas the experimental children test on all occasions within normal limits. The experimental group children appear to develop greater language competence at an earlier age than the controls. Experimental children appear more socially confident as infants and interact well with unfamiliar adults during early childhood.

We may think of programs of this type as improving the chances for positive achievement in disadvantaged children.

26

The Prenatal/Early Infancy Project

An Ecological Approach to Prevention of Developmental Disabilities

DAVID L. OLDS

In recent years we have witnessed increasing agreement that our nation's health strategy must be dramatically altered to emphasize disease prevention and health promotion. In the field of maternal and child health, there is an emerging belief that we have the scientific know-how to prevent some of the most devastating and costly problems of childhood. Prematurity and low birth weight, infant mortality, poor growth and nutrition, accidents, poisonings, certain illnesses, and some learning and psychosocial dysfunctions are among the major problems of infancy and early childhood that are considered preventable. Low birth weight (less than 5½ pounds) is of central importance because it poses the greatest threat to the life and health of infants. Two-thirds of all infant deaths occur in infants of low birth weight, and infants falling into this category are more likely than normal birth weight babies to be afflicted with mental retardation, birth defects, growth and developmental problems, blindness, autism, cerebral palsy, epilepsy, and child abuse, especially if they are reared in impoverished home environments (Richmond 1979; Sameroff & Chandler 1975). Investigations indicate that parental behavior plays an important role in the development of some of these difficulties, but the behavior of parents must be understood in terms of the overwhelming poverty, social disorganization, isolation, and stress with which many families must contend.

A number of strategies have been employed to address these problems by providing various supports to parents. They include comprehensive clinics for pregnant adolescents; nutritional supplementation programs for pregnant mothers at medical risk; early and extended contact between parents and newborns; mobile pediatric units for the urban poor; and parent education programs to encourage specific child rearing, safety, or health practices. Controlled studies of these interventions, while encouraging in some respects, have produced limited or contradictory results overall. Although the reasons for the mixed success of these programs vary, a major factor that needs to be considered in their interpretation is the extent to which their strategies altered the developmental context in which the family was trying to function. Most of the programs were based on the premise that the alteration of a single causative agent could improve the health or development of the child when, in fact, most of these problems are deeply embedded in interpersonal, familial, social, and economic contexts that in many ways overdetermine the emergence of undesirable outcomes.

Indeed, some have argued that the problems listed above are so inextricably interwoven into the fabric of our social and economic order that parent education or medical care in themselves can have little impact on reducing their incidence. Instead, their prevention will require major shifts in the distribution of income, the rates of unemployment, the incidence of racial and sex discrimination, and the availability of focused economic and social supports for families (Keniston 1977; McKinley 1979; National Academy of Sciences 1976). Most of these strategies, however, are outside the realm of health or human service professionals, are politically unacceptable at this time, and have unknown consequences for maternal and child health. As a short-term alternative to these long-range structural changes in society, we are currently investigating the effectiveness of a program that employs nurse home visitors and existing health and human services in an attempt to improve critical features of the prenatal and infancy environments that have been implicated in the etiology of the health and developmental problems enumerated above.

Known as the Prenatal/Early Infancy Project, the program is carried out in a semirural county in the Appalachian region of New York State. The heart of the program consists of nurse home visitation and the creation of informal and formal community support systems for families who are at risk for bearing and rearing children with the above-listed problems—families where first-time parents are either teenagers, single, or poor. In order to avoid creating a program that is stigmatized as being only for poor people or people with problems, the services are available to anyone in the community bearing a first baby. Active recruitment, however, focuses on families who are at risk. In our attempt to prevent health problems and to enhance the development of children born into these families, we have relied heavily on interrelated concepts: timing and ecology.

Beginning the program during pregnancy is considered crucial for its success. Home visitation starts sometime before the twenty-fourth week of pregnancy, with visits being made about twice a month, and continues through the second year of the baby's life, with less frequent visits as the child becomes older. We begin the program during pregnancy and continue it into infancy because these are considered highly labile phases in the life cycle of families during which the potential for helping (as well as harming) the child and family is unusually strong. From the standpoint of helping, it is our clinical judgment as well as the judgment of other investigators (Siegel et al. 1980) that beginning the program during pregnancy is important in terms of developing an effective caring relationship with parents. We reason that mothers are more likely to accept support when they are going through the profound and sensitive biological, psychological, and social changes produced by pregnancy. Parents are less likely to be defensive, we believe, if help is offered during pregnancy when all first-time parents, regardless of their income or personal situation, have questions and special needs. Offering help once the baby is born, on the other hand, may be interpreted as an indication that the service provider believes that parents have made mistakes or are incapable of caring for their children. And, if we are interested in preventing low birth weight or prematurity, assistance obviously must begin during pregnancy at the latest.

Precisely because the changes occurring during pregnancy are so delicate and profound, however, the potential for harming the fetus and family is equally great. In the biological realm, for example, a recent attempt to prevent prematurity and low birth weight by providing high protein nutritional supplements to medically high-risk indigent mothers during pregnancy actually increased the rate of premature delivery, neonatal death, and intrauterine growth retardation among babies born before the 37th week of gestation (Rush et al, 1980a, 1980b). This, of course, stresses the importance of systematically investigating the impact of even those services that may seem, on the face of it, to be helpful. In spite of the importance of initiating services during pregnancy, more is required than simply beginning early because the child health and developmental problems with which we are dealing are in many ways outgrowths of an environment that fails to provide sufficient support for families. It is here that the necessity of viewing these problems from an ecological perspective becomes evident.

In the Prenatal/Early Infancy Project (PEIP), parents are viewed as the most important environmental influence on the health and development of the child. Following the ecological theory of Bronfenbrenner (1979), however, we view the parent-child relationship as embedded in systems of informal social networks and formal relationships with health and human service providers, both of which can play powerful roles in supporting or undermining what goes on between parents and children. As we shall see, this theoretical conception has guided both the project and the investigation of the project's effectiveness.

From the standpoint of program content, the nurses are engaged in three basic activities that, in combination, form an ecological strategy for improving the conditions for pregnancy, birth, and early childrearing (Olds 1980). First, they provide parents with a home-based education program that focuses on factors that influence fetal and infant development and encourages sound prenatal health habits and child rearing behaviors. Second, in an attempt to create a more supportive informal environment for behavioral changes on the part of parents, they systematically involve "significant others" whom the mother would like to have participate in the home visits. And third, the nurses link families with other health and human services in the community so that the family's basic health and survival needs can be addressed. In the following sections these activities are elaborated upon so as to clarify how the program operates during pregnancy and after the newborn has arrived. In the final section, we discuss the role that ecological theory played in shaping the investigation of the service's effectiveness.

Nurse Home Visitation during Pregnancy

The two most basic goals for the pregnancy phase of the nurse home visitation program are to improve the mother's health habits so that better conditions exist for fetal development, and to enhance the family's psychological and social adjustment to pregnancy, birth, and early child rearing so that parents are better able to provide appropriate care for the young child. In order to achieve these objectives, it is essential that the nurses establish close communication and rapport with the mother-to-be and her family. Consequently, we have hired registered nurses who are parents themselves, are knowledgeable about the local community, and are compassionate, sensitive, and mature enough to give emotional support to others. Examples of supportive nursing behavior include responding to parents' concerns, helping them clarify their feelings, praising areas that parents are handling well, being aware of parents' special needs in times of stress, and encouraging them to develop their own problem-solving skills. We believe that to be truly supportive, the nurses must respect parents' values and not try to impose their own.

Parent Education

Evidence suggests that prematurity and low birth weight are associated with the mother's diet, use of alcohol and cigarettes, and psychological stress (Abramowitz and Kass 1966; Blau et al 1963). During the first and second trimesters, therefore, a major portion of the prenatal home-based education program focuses on improving maternal health habits with respect to these behaviors. To provide a motivational basis for mothers' following through with the nurses' recommendations regarding these health habits, mothers are given information on fetal development, the physiology of pregnancy, the stages of labor and delivery, and how each of these processes are related to the mother's behavior. We reasoned that by helping mothers understand how their behavior affects their health, their labor and delivery, and the health of their unborn children, the mothers would have a greater incentive to improve their health habits. The information is communicated in such a way that guilt and anxiety are minimized if a mother is unable to change.

Starting around the 28th week of pregnancy, the attention of parents usually begins to turn toward labor, delivery, and the early care of the newborn. Consistent with this, the nurse covers the following educational objectives during the last pregnancy visits: she sees to it that the mother and her support person are adequately prepared for the labor and delivery; that they understand the potential benefits of early and extended contact with the newborn (including rooming-in and breastfeeding) (Klaus and Kennell 1976); that they have gathered appropriate supplies for the baby; that they have selected a pediatrician; and that they are aware of some of the common tasks necessary for the physical care of their new family member. In addition, discussions are initiated with the mother and support person concerning normal infant behavior and individual differences in temperament, especially crying behavior. Also discussed toward the end of pregnancy are parents' plans for employment, school, contraceptive use, and the spacing of future children. The general approach is to provide anticipatory guidance so that the mother and the support person can make plans and rehearse strategies for coping with the newborn.

Relatives and Friends

A woman's prenatal health habits and competence in early child care have been related to the nature and quality of her relationships with "significant others" in her informal social environment (Cochran & Brassard 1979; McKinley 1972). Poor health habits, for example, are often woven into difficult family situations that have a direct bearing on a prospective mother's ability to alter her behavior: A woman whose husband is seeing other women may be anxious and smoke a great deal; one who has just lost her job may have no money for food; another whose own mother was heavily sedated during labor and delivery may lack maternal support for attending childbirth education classes or practicing breathing and relaxation techniques. For these reasons, a key aspect of the home visit program consists of involving family members or friends with whom mother feels very close. These may include her husband, boyfriend, mother, sister, or a friend. By including these individuals in the home visits, the nurse is able to impress upon them the importance of proper diet, rest, exercise, and regular prenatal care, as well as the dangers of smoking, drinking, and using drugs. Moreover, they are encouraged to accompany the mother-to-be to the obstetrician's office and childbirth education classes, to exercise and practice breathing and relaxation techniques with her, to act as coach during labor and delivery, and to help out with household responsibilities so that the mother does not overextend herself. With the help of these individuals, the women have a more supportive context for behavioral change.

During the last two months of pregnancy, the roles of fathers and other support people are reinforced even further. Their importance in providing the mother with physical comfort and emotional assurance during labor and delivery and their role in assisting with early child care are emphasized.

It is at this point that the enhancement of the mother's informal social support takes on a new dimension. All mothers are encouraged to identify one person living outside their own home whom they can turn to at any time during the day or night if they are having trouble with an irritable, inconsolable baby. We call this their "life-line" support and view it as especially important in preventing deterioration of the parent-child relationship under times of stress. By discussing these issues during pregnancy, before the baby is born, and by emphasizing how many parents are distressed with the care of an irritable, colicky newborn, we try to mimimize any implication that the mother is inadequate if she needs help in caring for the baby.

Linkages with Formal Services

In addition to enhancing the mother's informal support system, the nurse systematically links families with formal health and human service agencies. All parents are routinely encouraged to keep prenatal appointments and to enroll in childbirth education classes.

Families enrolled in PEIP receive their prenatal and well-child care either at private physicians' offices or at the local health department clinic, which is free to all families in the community. In order to strengthen the delivery of health care from these settings, the PEIP nurses send regular written reports containing information (such as nutritional inadequacies, health hazards, and emotional or social disturbances) gathered during visits that may help physicians and nurses provide more informed and sensitive care in the office. When necessary, office visits are arranged to discuss problem cases. During these visits, and through phone calls, the physician and nursing staff explain to the PEIP home visitor their medical care plan. With this information, the home visitor clarifies for the patient the physician's recommendations and thereby reinforces his or her advice. We think these nurse-mediated linkages between patient's home and physician's office result in better health care than could otherwise be expected because doctors' directives tend to be followed more consistently.

Because a significant number of families enrolled in our program live in isolated rural regions of the county, we have provided all families with a transportation back-up system so that they can have a means of getting to prenatal and well-child visits at the physician's office. We encourage the use of office and clinic-based health services because a number of investigators have linked the absence of these health services to a variety of health and developmental problems in children.

As noted above, many of the families enrolled in PEIP are preoccupied with pressing problems that interfere with mothers' developing appropriate health habits. Recognizing that such problems undermine the effects of their educational efforts and create special problems for the parents' later care of the infant, the nurses help their families find and use appropriate services in the community. A number of the parents in the program have been referred for help with mental health counseling; marital counseling; legal matters; diet planning and budgeting; diet supplementation from the Women, Infants, and Children (WIC) program; obtaining food stamps, Medicaid, and public assistance. In general, the nurses do not make the appointments for these services or serve as advocates for parents, as we are concerned that this may undermine the independence of parents, which we are attempting to foster. In order to facilitate parents' use of community services, rather than just providing them with phone numbers and names of service organizations, we have identified individuals within each of the organizations whom parents might contact. In this way we expect to help parents become more self-sufficient by personalizing the bureaucracy. However, when parents are believed to be mentally or emotionally impaired, or when referral agencies are not responding appropriately, the nurses do become actively involved in contacting agencies and in serving as advocates for the family.

In addition to helping families find community services to relieve the stresses of living in poverty or with strained family relations, the nurses also link parents with more specialized helping groups. Referrals are made to LaLeche to help mothers who decide to breastfeed, to CESAR, a local support group to aid mothers who are expecting to deliver by Caesarean section, and to Planned Parenthood to obtain inexpensive contraceptive supplies.

Nurse Home Visitation During Infancy

In spite of the joy that a newborn can bring to a family, the family situation is complicated by the birth, especially when the personal, social, and financial resources of parents are limited. The mother needs to recuperate and adapt to her new parenting role. The father or other support person must adjust to the new responsibilities of caring for a larger family at a time when he himself may feel particularly neglected. And, of course, the baby has very specific needs that must be met with insistent regularity.

Parent Education

The facilitation of parental adaptation that was begun toward the end of pregnancy is continued once the baby is born. The nurse pays a visit to the mother and baby in the hospital and again in the home about three days after they have returned from the hospital. In the hospital the nurse is present for the discharge examination so she can hear the physician's specific instructions. In this way, the nurse is able to reinforce the physician's advice with parents later. During the first home visit after birth, the nurse carries out a Brazelton Neonatal Assessment (Brazelton 1973), which serves as a vehicle for sensitizing parents to the baby's capabilities and ways of responding to the world. With this information about the baby, the nurse and family members can make plans for organizing the infant's environment to minimize distress and optimize the infant's development. The passive infant, for example, may need extra stimulation because he does not engage others readily; the irritable child who responds poorly to changes in his environment, on the other hand, may need to be protected from hoardes of well-wishing relatives and friends.

While emphasis is placed on the needs and characteristics of the infant, the mother's needs are addressed too. The nurse is continually aware of how the mother is coping with the infant's care and whether she is exhibiting any signs of post partum depression. Counselling about the resumption of sexual relations, birth control, schooling, and employment are among the topics covered by the nurse during the early months of life.

A large portion of the home visit time is devoted to helping parents with the physical care and feeding of the infant. The nurse demonstrate how to bathe the baby, treat diaper rash, and care for the umbilical cord and the circumcised prepuce, and they explain common newborn behaviors, how to manage common health problems, and the need for routine health care and immunization. As part of the curriculum concerning home and car safety, the nurses discuss such topics as the importance of using appropriate car seats and checking the crib to assure safe design. Mothers who breastfeed are given specific suggestions for making it a more enjoyable experience, while those who bottle feed are assisted with information on formula preparation, refrigeration, and so forth.

In the first few weeks of the newborn's life, home visits touch on the developmental accomplishments of the child, such as smiling and cooing to social stimuli, visual tracking, and orienting to sounds. Parents are encouraged to identify and respond to the infant's cues and to not worry about "spoiling" the child in these early months. As the child grows, parents are offered specific suggestions for activities that are likely to enhance development. Books and pamphlets describing such activities are provided and, surprisingly, are read by parents more frequently than we originally anticipated.

Beginning around the end of the first year of life, the content of the home visit sessions shifts to take into account the now mobile and talking toddler. Safety and educational needs take on new importance as the child begins to get into everything, to express his curiosity, and to talk. This is a period fraught with problems and potential. Not always knowing his limits, the child becomes a physical threat to himself; wanting to express his newly found autonomy, he becomes increasingly negative. So, in addition to helping parents with the child's changing nutritional needs and eating patterns, beginning toilet training, and common illnesses, the nurse assists them with strategies for baby-proofing the house, for handling temper tantrums, and for turning the child's potentially bothersome forays into kitchen cabinets into opportunities for learning. Parents are encouraged to turn daily events into times for teaching the names of things and how they work.

Involving Relatives and Friends

The early weeks after the arrival of the newborn can be particularly difficult extra for new mothers, especially if they are young, single, and lacking in financial resources. Under these circumstances, the support of fathers, grandmothers, other family members, and friends is crucial; without their involvement caring for the infant can be overwhelming. For these reasons, "significant others" continue to be invited to participate in the home visit sessions and to help solve particular problems that arise during this time.

If the father is an active participant, both parents are encouraged to make time for themselves alone, away from the baby, so that they may reestablish themselves as a couple. The mother also is encouraged to find several reliable baby sitters who might provide care for the infant if she decides to continue her education or employment or if she needs some time for herself. A well-organized system of child care is considered important for parents' ability to care for their child, so the nurses work with parents to identify persons who can fill this role. At the same time, however, parents are advised not to take advantage of these supportive individuals' good will by leaving their baby with them too frequently or by making too many other demands on them without reciprocating in some way.

Since it is almost impossible to arrange home visits so that fathers and other support persons can be present every time, specific visits have been identified for a minimum level of father or support person involvement. Around the fourth month of life, the home visitor arranges such a visit in which she concentrates on discussing infant temperament, early growth, and games that parents can play with the baby to enhance its development. Later, around the eighth month, the nurse arranges a special home visit in which she administers a questionnaire to help parents resolve differences they may have concerning disciplinary matters, encouraging independence, sex role training, and other issues of concern to them. During this visit parents relate how they themselves were brought up, the extent to which they want to raise their child the same way, how they would handle certain child rearing dilemmas, and why. This kind of process, it is believed, promotes open communication between partners and helps to resolve their differences on child rearing by encouraging them to anticipate conflicts and rehearse methods of dealing with them. Throughout the second year, fathers and other support persons are involved in at least two visits. At around the twelfth month, they are specifically invited to discuss the changing characteristics of the child and the difficulties these present for parents. At around the sixteenth month, they are invited again for a special session on negativism and the "terrible twos."

Linkages with Formal Services

As during pregnancy, a close working relationship with the physician's office is maintained. Regular reports are sent to the physician and frequent phone contacts are used to resolve problems related to the health and care of the baby. Likewise, difficulties affecting family life are addressed by referring families to the more specialized human service agencies in the community. The reduction of the stress associated with difficult family circumstances is thought to be important in preventing dysfunctions that lead to inadequate caregiving and maltreatment. By the time babies have reached their second year, these family difficulties have been addressed with the assistance of the nurse and other health and human service providers. Inevitably, however, some problems persist.

At two years of age, all children and families are referred to a locally established program that provides health and developmental screening and follow-up services for children and families. With the approval of parents, information on the child and the family is given to the screening program staff so that they can continue to help the preschoolers and parents until the children enter school.

An Ecologically Conceived Investigation

It is important to stress that the program just described was established as part of a major research effort to determine whether we can, indeed, prevent a whole host of health and developmental problems in children. We have attempted to go beyond simply determining whether the program works, however, by trying to determine whether specific program components are especially important, whether observed improvements in child health can be attributed to certain processes set in motion by the program, and whether certain families benefit more than others from the type of family support we have created. Moreover, by examining the interrelations among characteristics of the children, their families, and the ecological contexts in which they are living, we hope to gain a better understanding of important influences on the child.

In order to address these issues, 400 families (85 percent of whom are at risk) have been randomly assigned into four distinct service programs, three of which represent a subset of the total intervention described above. By comparing the mothers and children receiving these different services, we are able to determine the effectiveness of different components of the overall intervention.

The outcomes or dependent variables consist of critical aspects of the child's health and development that theoretically are likely to be affected by the nursing services (e.g., low birth weight, frequency of selected illnesses, developmental delays, and child abuse and neglect). In keeping with our overall theoretical framework, a number of additional variables have been measured at various levels of the ecological system in order to better understand the processes through which the program has imparted its effects. They consist of specific aspects of the environments that we have tried to affect: maternal health habits during pregnancy, parental child rearing practices, the level of informal support provided to mothers, parents' use of formal community services, and so forth. We hypothesize that the program will be effective to the extent that it is able to affect these processes positively.

Because we do not expect the services to be uniformly effective with all families, we also are examining a number of theoretically important characteristics of mothers and their families that may either affect the outcomes of the study or the mothers' ability to take advantage of the services provided. Specifically, we are looking at characteristics such as maternal health and psychological status before the services were provided, the level of pre-intervention social support available to mother, and certain constitutional and temperamental characteristics of the infant. In addition, we are carrying out a cost-benefit analysis to determine the extent to which the initial cost of the program is offset by reductions in later expenses for hospital care, emergency room visits, and special services for the handicapped.

Conclusion

Even though we have invested a great deal of thought in the design of this program, we have only a limited allegiance to it. The results of the project will be analyzed over the next several years, but it is inevitable that this strategy will have only limited success. Although we are optimistic about its effectiveness, certain outcomes and certain subpopulations are likely to be unaffected by the program. There are no miraculous solutions that can completely counteract the influence of families' living under oppressive circumstances for generation after generation. Although families' responses to the program are, on the whole, remarkably positive, variations in response exist. Common difficulties include home visits that are cancelled or simply not attended by parents, parental apathy about the material presented, differences between the values of the nurses and the individuals whom mothers rely on for informal help, and the absence of systematic social and economic supports for meeting families' basic necessities for survival. Moreover, there is a small but significant number of families who decline to enroll in the program—about 10 to 15 percent of those asked to join. Although a variety of reasons exist for nonparticipation, some of these families probably are at special risk, and we have not yet found a way of reaching them with this type of intervention.

This should give pause to those who wish to plunge into a full-scale programmatic initiative in this area. There is reason to be optimistic, but we have much to learn about the strategy before huge investments are made for services. Any serious consideration of an investment in home visiting should include a considerable investment in studying the strategy in settings different from the one described here so that it can be determined if the program will be successful, if it will produce any harmful effects, and if it can be improved.

Some workers have suggested that PEIP is so intensive that it is likely to be too expensive to carry out on a large scale. If we are successful in preventing just some prematurity and low birth weight, however, the long-range savings to society would be incalculable. Even in the short run the cost of dealing with these problems is staggering. In 1978, it cost over $500 per day to keep a premature newborn in a neonatal intensive care unit (Special Report, Robert Wood Johnson Foundation 1978), and it was not unheard of for the cost of a single sick neonate to exceed $100,000 (Grylack and Scanlon 1979). Just preventing admissions to neonatal ICUs alone would absorb a large portion of the costs of home visiting. This, of course, says nothing about the value of preventing lifetimes of human suffering and misery. In light of these human costs, and the possibility of our preventing them, how can we afford not to initiate more intervention research efforts in this area? Our chances for at least some success are good.

References

Abramowicz, M. & E. Kass. Pathogenesis and prognosis of prematurity. *New England Journal of Medicine* 166, 275:16–19.

Ainsworth, M. D. S. 1967. *Infancy in Uganda: Infant Care and the Growth of Love*. Baltimore: Johns Hopkins University Press.

Ainsworth, M. D. S. 1969. Object relations, dependency, and attachment: A theoretical review of the infant-mother relationship. *Child Development* 40:969–1025.

Ainsworth, M. D. S. 1973. The development of mother-infant attachment. In B. Caldwell & H. Ricciuti, eds., *Review of Child Development Research*, vol. 3. Chicago: University of Chicago Press.

Ainsworth, M. D. S. & S. M. V. Bell. 1969. Some contemporary patterns of mother-infant interaction in the feeding situation. In A. Ambrose, ed., *Stimulation in Early Infancy*. London: Academic Press.

Ainsworth, M. D. S. & S. M. V. Bell. 1970. Attachment, exploration, and separation: Illustrated by the behavior of one-year-olds in a strange situation. *Child Development* 41:49–67.

Ainsworth, M. D. S. & S. M. V. Bell. 1974. Mother-infant interaction and the development of competence. In K. Connolly & J. Bruner, eds., *The Growth of Competence*. New York: Academic Press.

Ainsworth, M. D. S., S. M. V. Bell, & D. M. Stayton. 1971. Individual differences in strange situation behavior of one year olds. In H. R. Schaffer, ed., *The Origins of Human Social Relations*. London: Academic Press.

Ainsworth, M. D. S., M. C. Blehar, E. Waters, & S. Wall. 1978. *Patterns of Attachment*. Hillsdale, N.J.: Erlbaum.

Ainsworth, M. D. S. & D. S. Wittig. 1969. Attachment and exploratory behavior of one year olds in a strange situation. In B. M. Foss, ed., *Determinants of Infant Behavior*, vol. 4. London: Methuen.

Alberman, E., M. Creasy, & C. Spicer. 1976. Maternal factors associated with fetal chromosomal anomalies in spontaneous abortions. *British Journal of Obstetrics and Gynaecology* 83:621–27.

Andrews, J. & J. McGarry. A community study of smoking in pregnancy. *Journal of Obstetrics and Gynaecology of the British Commonwealth* 79:1057–73.

Anderson, R. & J. F. Rosenblith. 1971. Sudden unexpected death syndrome: Early indicators. *Biology of the Neonate* 18:395–406.
Arend, R. A., F. L. Gove, & L. A. Sroufe. 1979. Continuity of early adaptation: From attachment in infancy to ego-resiliency and curiosity at age 5. *Child Development* 50:950–59.
Astrup, P., H. Olsen, D. Trolle, & K. Kieldsen. 1972. Effect of moderate carbon-monoxide exposure on fetal development. *Lancet* 2:1220–22.
Baer, M. Women workers and home responsibilities. 1954. *International Labor Review*, 69:338–55.
Bailey, R. The effects of maternal smoking on the infant birth weight. 1970. *New Zealand Journal of Medicine* 71:293–294.
Ban, P. L. & M. Lewis. 1974. Mothers and fathers, girls and boys: Attachment behavior in the one-year-old. *Merrill-Palmer Quarterly* 20:195–204.
Barnett, C. & R. Grobstein. 1974. Personal communication.
Barnett, C. R., P. H. Leiderman, R. Grobstein, & M. H. Klaus. 1970. Neonatal separation: The maternal side of interactional deprivation. *Pediatrics* 45:197–205.
Bates, E. 1979. *The Emergence of Symbols*. New York: Academic Press.
Bates, E. 1976. *Language and Context: The Acquisition of Pragmatics*. New York: Academic Press.
Bates, E., L. Camaioni, & V. Volterra. 1975. The acquisition of performatives prior to speech. *Merrill-Palmer Quarterly* 21:205–26.
Bateson, M. C. 1975. Mother-infant exchanges: The epigenesis of conversational interaction. In D. Aaronson and R. Rieber, eds., *Developmental Psycholinguistics and Communication Disorders*. Annals of N.Y. Academy of Science.
Bayley, N. 1970. Development of mental abilities. In P. H. Mussen, ed., *Carmichael's Manual of Child Psychology*, vol. 1. New York: Wiley.
Beckwith, L. & S. E. Cohen. 1978. Preterm birth: Hazardous obstetrical and postnatal events as related to caregiver-infant behavior. *Infant Behavior and Development* 1:403–12.
Bell, R. 1968. A reinterpretation of the direction of effects in studies of socialization. *Psychological Review* 75:81–95.
Belsky, J. 1980. A family analysis of parental influence on infant exploratory competence. In F. Pedersen, ed., *The Father-Infant Relationship: Observational Studies in a Family Context*. New York: Praeger Special Studies.
Belsky, J., M. Goode, & R. Most. 1980. Maternal stimulation and infant exploratory competence: Cross-sectional, correlational, and experimental analyses. *Child Development*, in press.

Bergman, A. B. & L. A. Wiesner. 1976. Relationship of passive cigarette-smoking to sudden infant death syndrome. *Pediatrics* 58:665–68.

Berlyne, D. E. 1958. The influence of the albedo and complexity of stimuli on visual fixation in the human infant. *British Journal of Psychology*, 49:315–18.

Berman, P. W. 1976. Social context as a determinant of sex differences in adults' attraction to infants. *Developmental Psychology* 12:365–66.

Bernhard, P. 1948. Der einfluss des zigarettenrauchers auf die schwangere frau. *Zentrablatt fur Gynakologie* 70:18.

Biller, H. B. & D. L. Merredith. 1974. *Father Power*. New York: McKay.

Blau, A., B. Slabb, K. Easton, J. Welkowitz, J. Spingarn & J. Cohen 1963. The psychogenic etiology of premature births: A preliminary report. *Psychosomatic Medicine* 30:201–11.

Blehar, M. 1974. Anxious attachment and defensive reactions associated with day care. *Child Development* 45:683–92.

Block, J. H. & J. Block. 1979. The role of ego-control and ego-resiliency in the organization of behavior. In W. A. Collins, ed., *Minnesota Symposia on Child Psychology*, vol. 11. Hillsdale, N.J.: Erlbaum.

Bornstein, M. H. 1976. Infants are trichromats. *Journal of Experimental Child Psychology* 21:425–45.

Bowlby, J. 1951. *Maternal Care and Mental Health*. Geneva: World Health Organization.

Bowlby, J. 1958. The nature of the child's tie to his mother. *International Journal of Psychoanalysis* 39:350–373.

Bowlby, J. 1969. *Attachment and loss*. Vol. 1. *Attachment*. New York: Basic Books.

Brachfeld, S. & S. Goldberg. 1978. Parent-infant interaction: Effects of newborn medical status on free play at 8 and 12 months. Presented at the meeting of the Southeastern Conference on Human Development, April. Atlanta.

Brazelton, T. B. 1973. *Neonatal Behavioral Assessment Scale*. London: Heineman.

Brazelton, T. B., B. Kowsolwski, & M. Main. 1974. The origins of reciprocity: The early mother-infant interaction. In M. Lewis & L. Rosenblum, eds., *The Effect of the Infant on Its Caregiver*. New York: Wiley.

Brennan, W. M., E. W. Ames, & R. W. Moore. 1966. Age differences in infants' attention to patterns of different complexities. *Science* 151:354–56.

Bridges, K. M. B. 1933. A study of social development in early infancy. *Child Development* 4:36–49.

Bronfenbrenner, U. 1970. *Two Worlds of Childhood: U.S. and U.S.S.R.* New York: Russell Sage Foundation.

Bronfenbrenner, U. 1974. Developmental research, public policy, and the ecology of childhood. *Child Development* 45:1–5.
Bronfenbrenner, U. 1975. Is early intervention effective? In M. Guttentag and E. Stevening, eds., *Handbook of Evaluation Research*, vol. 2. Beverly Hills, Calif: Sage Publications.
Bronfenbrenner, U. 1977. Toward an experimental ecology of human development. *American Psychologist* 32:513–31.
Bronfenbrenner, U. 1979. *The Ecology of Human Development: Experiments by Nature and Design*. Cambridge: Harvard University Press.
Brookhart, J. & E. Hock. 1976. The effects of experimental context and experiential background on infants' behavior toward their mothers and a stranger. *Child Development* 47:333–40.
Brooks-Gunn, J. & M. Lewis. 1976. Infants' responses to strangers: Midget, adult, and child. *Child Development* 47:323–32.
Brown, R. & J. Bakeman. 1979. Relationships of human mothers with their infants during the first year of life. In R. W. Bell & W. P. Smotherman, eds. *Maternal influences on early behavior*. Hollis-wood, New York: Spectrum.
Bruner, J. 1977. Early social interaction and language acquisition. In H. R. Schaffer, ed., *Studies in Mother-Infant Interaction*. New York: Academic Press.
Bruner, J. S. 1973. Organization of early skilled action. *Child Development* 44:1–11.
Bühler, C. 1930. *The First Year of Life*. New York: John Day.
Buncher, C. 1969. Cigarette smoking and duration of pregnancy. *American Journal of Obstetrics and Gynaecology* 103:942–46.
Butler, N. & E. Alberman. 1969. Perinatal Problems. *Second Report of the 1958 British Perinatal Mortality Survey*. Edinburgh: Livingstone.
Butler, N. & H. Goldstein. 1974. Smoking in pregnancy and subsequent child development. *British Journal of Medicine* 4:573–75.
Caldwell, B. M., C. M. Wright, A. S. Honig, & J. Tannerbaum. 1970. Infant care and attachment. *American Journal of Orthopsychiatry* 40:397–412.
Campbell, A. 1936. The effect of excessive cigarette smoking on maternal health. *American Journal of Obstetrics and Gynaecology* 31:502–8.
Chase, W. P. 1937. Color vision in infants. *Journal of Experimental Psychology* 20:203–222.
Child Care Data and Materials. 1974. Committee on Finance, United States Senate (Committee print). Washington, D.C.: Government Printing Office.
Clarke-Stewart, K. A. 1973. Interactions between mothers and their young children: Characteristics and consequences. *Monographs of*

the Society for Research in Child Development 38:6–7. Serial no. 153.

Cleaves, W. T. & P. C. Rosenblatt. 1977. Intimacy between adults and children in public places. Paper presented at the biennial meeting of the Society for Research in Child Development, March. New Orleans.

Coates, B., E. P. Anderson, & W. W. Hartup. 1972. Interrelations in the attachment behavior of human infants. *Developmental Psychology* 6(2):218–30.

Cochran, M. 1977. A comparison of group day and family child-rearing patterns in Sweden. *Child Development* 48:702–7.

Cochran, M. & J. Brassard. 1979. Child development and personal social networks. *Child Development* 50:601–16.

Cohen, L. B. & N. F. Caputo. 1978. Instructing infants to respond to perceptual categories. Paper presented at the meeting of the Midwestern Psychological Association, May 1978, Chicago.

Cohen, L. B., J. S. DeLoache, & R. Pearl. 1977. An examination of interference effects in infants' memory for faces. *Child Development* 48:88–96.

Cohen, L. B., J. S. DeLoache, & M. S. Strauss. 1979. Infant perceptual development. In J. D. Osofsky, ed., *Handbook of Infant Development*. New York: Wiley.

Cohen, L. B. & E. R. Gelber. 1975. Infant visual memory. In L. Cohen & P. Salapatek, eds., *Infant Perception: From Sensation to Cognition, vol 1. Basic Visual Processes*. New York: Academic Press.

Cohen, L. B., & M. S. Strauss. 1979. Concept acquisition in the human infant. *Child Development* 50:419–24.

Comstock, G., F. Shah, M. Meyer, & H. Abbey. 1971. Low birth weight and neonatal mortality rate related to maternal smoking and socioeconomic status. *American Journal of Obstetrics and Gynaecology* 111:53–59.

Condon, W. S. & L. W. Sander. 1974. Neonate movement is synchronized with adult speech: Interactional participation and language acquisition. *Science* 183:99–101.

Cope, I., P. Lancaster, & L. Stevens. 1973. Smoking in pregnancy. *Medical Journal of Australia* 1:673–77.

Cornell, E. H. 1974. Infants' discrimination of faces following redundant presentations. *Journal of Experimental Child Psychology* 18:98–106.

Cruickshank, R. M. 1941. The development of visual size constancy in early infancy. *Journal of Genetic Psychology* 58:327–51.

Davie, R., N. Butler, & H. Goldstein. 1972. *From Birth to Seven*. London: William Clowes.

Davies, D., O. Gray, P. Ellwood, & M. Abernethy. 1976. Cigarette smoking in pregnancy. *Lancet* 1:385–87.

Denson, R., J. Nanson, & M. McWatters. 1975. Hyperkinesis and maternal smoking. *Canadian Psychological Association Journal* 20:183–87.

DeSouza, S., R. John, & B. Richards. 1976. Studies on the effect of pre-eclamptic toxaemia on placental weight and on head size and birth weight of the newborn. *British Journal of Obstetrics and Gynaecology* 83:292–98.

DiVitto, B. & S. Goldberg. 1979. The development of early parent-infant interaction as a function of newborn medical status. In T. Field, A. Sostek, S. Goldberg, & H. H. Shuman, eds., *Infants Born at Risk*. Holliswood, N.Y.: Spectrum.

Dobbing, J. 1975. Human brain development and its vulnerability. In Mead Johnson Symposium on Perinatal and Developmental Medicine, No. 6: *Biological and Clinical Aspects of Brain Development* 3–12.

Dobson, V., D. Y. Teller, C. P. Lee, & B. Wade. 1978. A behavioral method for efficient screening of visual acuity in young infants. *Investigative Ophthalmology and Visual Science* 17:1142–50.

Donovan, J. 1977. Randomised controlled trial of antismoking advice in pregnancy. *British Journal of Society for Preventive Medicine* 31:6–12.

Doyle, A. 1975. Infant development in day care. *Developmental Psychology* 11:655–56.

Doyle, A. & K. Somers. 1977. The effects of group and family day care on infant attachment. Unpublished manuscript, Concordia University, Montreal.

Drillien, C. M. 1964. *The Growth and Development of the Prematurely Born Infant*. Baltimore: Williams & Wilkins.

Dunn, H., S. McBurner, S. Ingram, S. & C. Hunter. 1976. Maternal cigarette smoking during pregnancy and the child's subsequent development: I. Physical growth to the age of 6½years. *Canadian Journal of Public Health* 67:499–505.

Dunn, H., S. McBurner, S. Ingram, & C. Hunter. 1977. Maternal cigarette smoking during pregnancy and the child's subsequent development: II. Neurological and intellectual maturation to the age of 6½ years. *Canadian Journal of Public Health* 68:43–50.

Dunn, L. M., L. T. Chun, D. C. Crowell, L. M. Dunn, L. G. Alevy, & E. R. Yachel. 1976. *Peabody Early Education Kit*. Circle Pines, Minn.: American Guidance Service.

Eckerman, C. O., J. L. Whatley, & S. L. Kutz. 1975. Growth of social play with peers during the second year of life. *Developmental Psychology* 11:42–49.

Edwards, C. P. & B. B. Whiting. 1966. Dependency in dyadic contexts: New meaning for an old construct. Paper presented to the Eastern Psychological Association, April 1976, New York.

Eibel-Eibesfeldt, I. 1970. *Ethology: The Biology of Behavior.* New York: Holt, Rhinehart & Winston.

Eimas, P. D., E. R. Siqueland, P. Jusczyk, & J. Vigorito. 1971. Speech perception in infants. *Science* 171:303–6.

Epstein, A. S. 1979. The stability of behavior: I. On predicting most of the people much of the time. *Journal of Personality and Social Psychology* 37:1098–1126.

Epstein, A. S. & N. Radin. 1975. Motivational components related to father behavior and cognitive functioning in preschoolers. *Child Development* 46:831–839.

Erikson, E. H. 1963. *Childhood and Society.* 2d ed. New York: Norton.

Escalona, S. 1968. *The Roots of Individuality.* Chicago: Aldine.

Essenberg, J., J. Schwind, & A. Peters. 1940. The effects of nicotine and cigarette smoke on pregnant female albino rats and their offspring. *Journal of Clinical Laboratory Medicine* 25:708–717.

Etaugh, C. 1974. Effect of maternal employment on children: A review of recent research. *Merrill-Palmer Quarterly* 20:71–98.

Fagan, J. F. 1973. Infants' delayed recognition memory and forgetting. Journal of Experimental Child Psychology 16:424–50.

Fagan, J. F. 1974. Infants' recognition of invariant features of faces. *Child Development* 47:627–38.

Fagan, J. F. 1977. An attention model of infant recognition. *Child Development* 48:345–59.

Fantz, R. L. 1961. The origin of form perception. *Scientific American* 204(5):66–72.

Fantz, R. L. 1963. Pattern vision in newborn infants. *Science* 140:296–97.

Fantz, R. L. 1964. Visual experience in infants: Decreased attention to familiar patterns relative to novel ones. *Science* 146:668–70.

Fantz, R. L. 1965. Visual perception from birth as shown by pattern selectivity. *Annals of the New York Academy of Science* 118:793–814.

Fantz, R., J. Fagan, & S. Miranda. 1975. Early visual selectivity. In L. Cohen & P. Salapatek, eds., *Infant Perception: From Sensation to Cognition*, vol. 1. *Basic visual Processes.* New York: Academic Press.

Fantz, R. L. & S. Nevis. 1967. Pattern preferences and perceptual-cognitive development in early infancy. *Merrill-Palmer Quarterly* 13:77–108.

Fantz, R. L., J. M. Ordy, & M. S. Udelt. 1962. Maturation of pattern vision in infants during the first six months. *Journal of Comparative and Physiological Psychology* 55:907–17.

Farran, D. & C. Ramey. 1977. Infant day care and attachment behaviors toward mothers and teachers. *Child Development* 48:1112–16.

Fein, G. G. 1969. Echoes from the nursery: Piaget, Vygotsky, and the relationship between language and play. *New Directions for Child Development: Fact, Fiction and Fantasy in Childhood* 6:1–14.

Fein, G. G. & N. Apfel. 1979. The development of play: Style, structure, and situations. *Genetic Psychology Monographs* 99:231–50.
Feldman, S. & M. Ingham, 1975. Attachment behavior: A validation study in two age groups. *Child Development* 46:319–30.
Fenson, L., J. Kagan, R. B. Kearsley, & P. R. Zelazo. 1976. The developmental progression of manipulative play in the first two years. *Child Development* 47:232–36.
Fenson, L. & D. S. Ramsey. 1980. Decentration and integration of the child's play in the second year. *Child Development* 51:171–78.
Field, T. M. 1977a. Effects of early separation, interactive deficits, and experimental manipulations on infant-mother face-to-face interaction. *Child Development* 48:763–71.
Field, T. M. 1977b. Maternal stimulation during infant feeding. *Developmental Psychology* 13:539–40.
Field, T. M., N. Hallock, G. Ting, J. Dempsey, C. Dabiri, & H. H. Shumann. 1978. A first-year follow-up of high-risk infants: Formulating a cumulative risk index. *Child Development* 49:163–77.
Fowler, W. & N. Khan. 1974, 1975. The development of a prototype infant and child day care center in metropolitan Toronto. Ontario Institute for Studies in Education, Year III Progress Report, December 1974; Year IV Progress Report, December 1975.
Frazier, T., G. Tavis, H. Goldstein, & I. Goldbers. 1961. Cigarette smoking and prematurity: A prospective study. *American Journal of Obstetrics and Gynaecology* 81:988–96.
Freedle, R. & M. Lewis. 1977. Prelinguistic conversations. In M. Lewis and L. A. Rosenblum, eds., *Interaction, Conversation, and the Development of Language*. New York: Wiley.
Freud, S. 1961. *Civilization and Its Discontents*. New York: Norton.
Garn, S., H. Shaw, & K. McCabe. 1977. Relative effect of smoking and other variables on size of newborn. Lancet 2:667.
Garvey, C. 1974. Some properties of social play. *Merrill-Palmer Quarterly* 20:163–180.
Gennser, G., K. Marsal, & B. Brantmark. 1975. Maternal smoking and fetal breathing movements. *American Journal of Obstetrics and Gynaecology* 123:861–67.
Gerwitz, J. 1969. Mechanisms of social learning: Some roles of stimulation and behavior in early human development. In D. Goslin, ed., *Handbook of Socialization Theory and Research*. Chicago: Rand McNally.
Ginsburg, H. & B. Koslowski. 1976. Cognitive development. *Annual Review of Psychology* 27:29–61.
Goldberg, S. & M. Lewis. 1969. Play behavior in the year-old infant: Early sex differences. *Child Development* 40:21–31.
Golden, M. & B. Birns. 1976. Social class and infant intelligence. In M. Lewis, ed., *Origins of Intelligence*. New York: Plenum.

Golden, M., L. Rosenbluth, M. Grossi, H. Policare, H. Freeman, & E. Brownlee. 1978. *The New York City Infant Day Care Study*. New York: Medical and Health Research Association of New York City.
Goldfarb, W. 1943. The effects of early institutional care on adolescent personality. *Journal of Experimental Education* 12:106–129.
Goren, C. 1975. Form perception, innate form preferences and visually-mediated head turning in human newborns. Paper presented at the meeting of the Society for Research in Child Development, April 1975, Denver.
Goslin, D. A., ed. 1969. *Handbook of Socialization Theory and Research*. Chicago: Rand McNally.
Goujard, J., C. Rumeau, & D. Schwartz. 1975. Smoking during pregnancy, stillbirth and abruptio placentae. *Biomedica* 23:20–22.
Graham, F. 1956. Behavioral differences between normal and traumatic newborns: Test procedures. *Psychological Monographs* 70, no. 427.
Graham, H. 1976. Smoking in pregnancy: The attitudes of expectant mothers. *Society for Scientific Medicine* 10:399–405.
Greenberg, M. & N. Morris. 1974. Engrossment: The newborn's impact upon the father. *American Journal of Orthopsychiatry* 44:520–531.
Greenberg, M., D. Rosenberg, & J. Lind. 1973. First mothers rooming-in with their newborns: Its impact upon the mother. *American Journal of Orthopsychiatry* 43:783–788.
Greenberg, P. & B. Epstein. 1973. *Bridges to Reading*. Morristown, N.J.: General Learning Corp.
Griffiths, R. 1954. *The Abilities of Babies: A Study in Mental Measurement*. New York: McGraw-Hill.
Grylack, L. J. & J. W. Scanlon. 1979. Maternal and newborn health at Columbia Hospital for Women. *Urban Health*, September, 49–52.
Guilford, J. P. 1967. *The Nature of Human Intelligence*. New York: McGraw-Hill.
Gunther, M. 1955. Instinct and the nursing couple. *The Lancet* 1:575.
Gunther, M. 1961. Infant behavior at the breast. In B. Foss, ed., *Determinants of Infant Behavior*. London: Methuen and Co., 37–44.
Haddon, W., R. Nesbitt, & R. Garcia. 1961. Smoking and pregnancy: Carbon monoxide in blood during gestation and at term. *Obstetrics and Gynaecology* 18:262–67.
Halliday, M. 1979. One child's protolanguage. In M. Bullova, ed., *Before Speech: The Beginning of Interpersonal Communication*. New York: Cambridge University Press.
Handbook of Labor Statistics. 1976. U.S. Department of Labor, Bureau of Labor Statistics.
Harding, C. G. & R. M. Golinkoff. 1979. The origins of intentional vocalization in prelinguistic infants. *Child Development* 50:33–40.
Harding, C. G. & R. M. Golinkoff. 1980. Preverbal communication:

The role of cognitive development and maternal style. Paper presented at the Second International Conference on Infant Studies, April, 1980, New Haven, Conn.

Harlow, H. F. 1969. Age-mate or peer affectional system. In D. S. Lehrman, R. A. Hinde, & E. Shaw, eds., *Advances in the Study of Behavior*, vol. 2. New York: Academic Press.

Hart, H. L. A. 1961. *The Concept of Law*. Oxford: Oxford University Press.

Haskins, R., N. W. Finkelstein, & D. J. Stedman. 1978. Effects of infant and preschool stimulation programs on high-risk children: Intelligence, social behavior, and health. *Pediatric Annals* 7:123–44.

Haviland, J. & M. Lewis. 1976. Infants' greeting patterns to strangers. *Research Bulletin 76–2*. Princeton, N.J.: Educational Testing Service.

Heathers, G. 1955. Emotional dependence and independence in nursery school play. *Journal of Genetic Psychology* 87:37–57.

Hebb, D. O. 1946. On the nature of fear. *Psychological Review* 53:259–76.

Hebb, D. O. 1949. *The Organization of Behavior*. New York: Wiley.

Heber, R., H. Garber, D. Harrington, C. Hoffman, & C. Falender. 1972. *Rehabilitation of Families at Risk for Mental Retardation*. Rehabilitation Research and Training Center in Mental Retardation. Madison: University of Wisconsin.

Hellman, J., H. Johnson, W. Tolles, & E. Jones. 1961. Some factors affecting fetal heart rate. *American Journal of Obstetrics and Gynaecology* 82:1055–63.

Herriot, A., W. Bollewicz, & F. Hythens. 1962. Cigarette smoking in pregnancy. *Lancet* 1:771–73.

Hersler, L., J. Richmond, & A. Moore. 1963. Maternal behavior in sheep and goats. In H. Rheingold, ed., *Maternal Behavior in Mammals*. New York: Wiley.

Hill, P. M. & L. M. Nicolich. 1979. Pretend play and patterns of cognition in Down's syndrome children. Unpublished paper, Rutgers University.

Hinde, R. A. 1971. Development of social behavior. In A. M. Schrier & F. Stollnitz, eds., *Behavior of Nonhuman Primates: Modern Research Trends*, vol. 3. New York: Academic Press.

Hock, E. 1976. *Alternative approaches to child-rearing and their effects on the mother-infant relationship*. Columbus, Ohio: Ohio State University and Ohio Agricultural Research and Development Centers. ERIC Document Reproduction Service No. ED 122–943.

Hoffman, L. M. 1974. Effect of maternal employment on the child—a review of the research. *Developmental Psychology* 10:204–8.

Howell, M. C. 1974. Employed mothers and their families I, II. *Pediatrics* 52:252–63, 327–43.

Hunt, J. McV. 1961. *Intelligence and Experience.* New York: Ronald Press.

Järvinen, P. & K. Österlund. 1963. Effect of smoking during pregnancy on the fetus, placenta, and delivery. *Arr. Paediat. Fenniae* 9, 18–26.

Jones, K. L., D. W. Smith, A. Streissguth, & N. Myrianthopoulos. 1974. Outcome in offspring of chronic alcoholic women. *Lancet* 1:1076–78.

Jones, P. 1975. Smoking and pregnancy. *Nursing Times* 71:2038–39.

Kagan, J., R. Kearsley, & P. Zelazo. 1976. The effects of infant day care on psychological development. Paper presented at the meeting of the American Association for the Advancement of Science, February 1976, Boston.

Kaminski, M., C. Rumpao, & D. Schwartz. 1978. Alcohol consumption in pregnant women and the outcome of pregnancy. *Alcoholism: Clinical and Experimental Research* 2:155–163.

Kaplan, E. & G. Kaplan. 1971. The pre-linguistic child. In J. Elliot, ed., *Human Development and Cognitive Processes.* New York: Holt, Rinehart and Winston.

Karnes, M. B. 1973. *GOAL Program: Mathematical Concepts.* Springfield, Mass.: Milton-Bradley.

Karnes, M. B., & J. Teska. 1975. The effects of early intervention programs. In J. Gallagher, ed., *The Applications of Child Development Research with Exceptional Children.* Reston, Va: Council for Exceptional Children.

Keniston, K. 1977. *All Our Children: The American Family Under Pressure.* New York: Carnegie Corporation.

Kennell, J., R. Jeranld, H. Wolfe, D. Chester, N. Kreger, W. McAlpine, M. Steffa, & M. Klaus. 1974. Maternal behavior one year after early and extended post-partum contact. *Developmental Medicine and Child Neurology* 16:172–179.

Kennell, J. H. & M. H. Klaus. 1976. Caring for parents of a premature or sick infant. In M. H. Klaus & J. H. Kennell, eds., *Maternal-Infant Bonding.* St. Louis: Mosby.

Klaus, M., R. Jeranld, N. Kreger, W. McAlpine, M. Steffa, & J. Kennel. 1972. Maternal attachment—importance of the first post-partum days. *New England Journal of Medicine* 286:460–63.

Klaus, M. & J. Kennell, 1976. *Maternal-Infant Bonding.* St. Louis: Mosby.

Klaus, M. H., J. H. Kennell, N. Plumb, & S. Zuehlke. 1970. Human maternal behavior at the first contact with her young. *Pediatrics* 46:187–92.

Klein, J., Z. Stein, M. Susser, & D. Warburton. 1977. Smoking: A risk factor for spontaneous abortion. *New England Journal of Medicine* 297:793–96.

Klopfer, P. 1971. Mother love! What turns it on? *American Scientist* 49:404–7.

Kohr, R. L. & P. A. Games. 1974. Robustness of the analysis of variance, the Welch procedure and a box procedure to heterogeneous variances. *The Journal of Experimental Education* 43:61–69.

Kotelchuck, M. 1976. The infant's relationship to the father: Experimental evidence. In M. E. Lamb, ed., *The Role of the Father in Child Development*. New York: Wiley.

Kullander, S. & B. Källen. 1971. A prospective study of smoking and pregnancy. *Acta Obstet. Gynec. Scand.* 50:83–94.

Lally, R. 1973. The family development research program. Progress report. Mimeographed. Syracuse, N.Y.: Syracuse University.

Lally, R. 1974. The family development research program. Progress report. Mimeographed. Syracuse, N.Y.: Syracuse University.

Lamb, M. E. 1975a. Fathers: Forgotten contributors to child development. *Human Development* 18:245–66.

Lamb, M. E. 1975b. Infants, fathers, and mothers: Interaction at 8-months-of-age in the home and in the laboratory. Paper presented at the convention of the Eastern Psychological Association, April 1975, New York.

Lamb, M. E. 1975c. Infant attachment to mothers and fathers. Paper presented at the biennial meeting of the Society for Research in Child Development, April 1975, Denver.

Lamb, M. E. 1976a. Effects of stress and cohort on mother- and father-infant interaction. *Developmental Psychology* 12:435–43.

Lamb, M. E. 1976b. Interactions between two-year-olds and their mothers and fathers. *Psychological Reports* 38:447–50.

Lamb, M. E. 1976c. The role of the father: An overview. In M. E. Lamb, ed., *The Role of the Father in Child Development*. New York: Wiley.

Lamb, M. E. 1976d. Twelve-month-olds and their parents: Interaction in a laboratory playroom. *Developmental Psychology* 12:237–44.

Lamb, M. E. 1976e. Interactions between eight-month-old children and their fathers and mothers. In M. E. Lamb, ed., *The Role of the Father in Child Development*. New York: Wiley.

Lamb, M. E. 1977a. Father-infant and mother-infant interaction in the first year of life. *Child Development* 48:167–81.

Lamb, M. E. 1977b. The development of mother-infant and father-infant attachments in the second year of life. *Developmental Psychology* 13:637–48.

Lamb, M. E. 1977c. Development and function of parent-infant relationships in the first two years of life. Paper presented at the biennial meeting of the Society for Research in Child Development, March, New Orleans.

Lamb, M. E. 1977d. The effects of ecological variables on parent-infant interaction. Paper presented at the biennial meeting of the Society for Research in Child Development, March, New Orleans.

Lamb, M. E. 1977e. A reexamination of the infant social world. *Human Development* 20:65–85.

Landesman-Dwyer, S., L. Keller, & A. Streissguth. 1978. Naturalistic observations of newborns: Effects of maternal alcohol intake. *Alcoholism: Clinical and Experimental Research*, 2:171–77.

Lang, R. 1974. Personal communication.

Lee, L. C. 1973. Social encounters of infants: The beginnings of popularity. Paper presented to the International Society for the Study of Behavioural Development, Ann Arbor, Michigan.

Leiderman, P. H. & M. J. Seashore, 1975. Mother-infant separation: Some delayed consequences. In *Parent-Infant Interaction*. CIBA Foundation Symposium, no. 33. New York: Elsevier.

Leifer, A. D., P. H. Leiderman, C. R. Barnett, & J. A. Williams. 1972. Effects of mother-infant separation on maternal attachment behavior. *Child Development* 43:1203-18.

Levine, J. A. 1977. *Who will raise the children? New Options for Fathers (and Mothers)*. New York: Lippincott.

Lewis, J. 1975. Family development center: A demonstration project. Unpublished manuscript, Family Service Agency, San Francisco.

Lewis, M. & P. Ban. 1971. Stability of attachment behavior: A transformational analysis. Paper presented at a symposium on Attachment: Studies in Stability and Change at the meetings of the Society for Research in Child Development, April 1971, Minneapolis.

Lewis, M. & J. Brooks-Gunn. 1975. Infants' social perception: A constructivist view. In L. Cohen & P. Salapatek, eds., *Infant Perception: From Sensation to Cognition*, vol. 2. New York: Academic press.

Lewis, M. & S. Goldberg. 1969. Perceptual-cognitive development in infancy: A generalized expectancy model as a function of the mother-infant relationship. *Merrill-Palmer Quarterly* 15:81–100.

Lewis, M. & L. A. Rosenblum, eds. 1974. *Effect of the Infant on Its Caregivers*. New York: Wiley.

Lewis, M. & L. A. Rosenblum, eds. 1975. *Friendship and Peer Relations*. New York: Wiley.

Lewis, M. & M. Weinraub. 1974. Sex of parent X sex of child: Socioemotional development. In R. C. Friedman, R. M. Richart & R. L. Van de Wiele, eds., *Sex Differences in Behavior*. New York: Wiley.

Lewis, M. & M. Weinraub. 1976. The father's role in the infant's social network. In M. E. Lamb, ed., *The Role of the Father in Child Development*. New York: Wiley.

Lewis, M., G. Young, J. Brooks, & L. Michalson. 1975. The beginning of friendship. In M. Lewis & L. A. Rosenblum, eds., *Friendship and Peer Relations*. New York: Wiley.

Ling, B. C. 1941. Form discrimination as a learning cue in infants. *Comparative Psychology Monographs* 17(2, Whole No. 86).

Lipsitt, L. P. 1976. Developmental psychobiology comes of age: A discussion. In L. P. Lipsitt, ed., *Developmental Psychobiology: The Significance of Infancy*. Hillsdale, N.J.: Lawrence Erlbaum Associates.

Lipsitt, L. P., W. Q. Sturner, & P. M. Burke. 1979. Perinatal indicators and crib death. *Infant Behavior and Development* 2:325–329.

Loevinger, J. 1976. *Ego Development*. London: Jossey-Bass.

Longo, L. 1976. Carbon monoxide effects of oxygenation of the fetus in utero. *Science* 194:523–525.

Lorenz, K. Z. 1943. Die angeborenen Lormen Moglicker Erfahrung. *Zeitschrift fur Tierpsychologie* 5:235–409.

Lowe, C. R. 1959. Effect of mothers' smoking habits on birth weight of their children. *British Medical Journal* 2:673–676.

Lund, J., V. Vuorenkoski, & O. Wasz-Hoeckert. 1973. The effect of cry to stimulus on the temperature of the lactating breast primipara: A thermographic study. In N. Morris, ed., *Psychosomatic Medicine in Obstetrics and Gynaecology*. Basel, Switzerland: S. Karger.

Lynn, D. B. 1974. *The Father: His Role in Child Development*. Monterey, Calif.: Brooks/Cole.

Lynn, D. B. & A. R. Cross. 1974. Parent preference of preschool children. *Journal of Marriage and the Family* 36:555–59.

McBryde, A. 1951. Compulsory rooming-in in the ward and private newborn service at Duke Hospital. *Journal of the American Medical Association* 45:625.

McCall, R. 1977. Challenges to a science of developmental psychology. *Child Development* 48:333–44.

McCall, R. B. 1974. Exploratory manipulation and play in the human infant. *Monographs of the Society for Research in Child Development* 39, no. 155.

McCall, R. B. 1977. Stages in mental development during the first two years. Paper presented at the biennial meeting of the Society for Research in Child Development, March 1977, New Orleans.

McCall, R. B., D. H. Eichorn, & P. S. Hogarty. 1977. Transitions in early mental development. *Monographs of the Society for Research in Child Development* 42, no. 171.

McCall, R. B., C. B. Kennedy, & C. Dodds. 1977. The interfering effect of distracting stimuli on the infant's memory. *Child Development* 48:79–87.

McGurk, H. 1972. Infant discrimination of orientation. *Journal of Experimental Child Psychology* 14:151–164.

McKinlay, J. B. 1979. Epidemiological and political determinants of social policies regarding the public health. *Social Science and Medicine* 13A:541–558.

McKinley, J. 1973. Social networks, lay consultation, and help-seeking behavior. *Social Forces* 15:275–292.
Mahler, M. S. 1975. *The Psychological Birth of the Human Infant*. New York: Basic Books.
Main, M. 1973. Exploration, play, and cognitive functioning as related to child-mother attachment. Unpublished doctoral dissertation. Baltimore: Johns Hopkins University.
Main, M. 1977. Analysis of a peculiar form of reunion behavior seen in some day-care children: Its history and sequelae in children who are home-reared. In R. Webb, ed., *Social Development in Childhood: Daycare Programs and Research*. Baltimore: Johns Hopkins University Press.
Main, M. 1977. Sicherheit und Wissen. In K. E. Grossman, ed., *Entwicklung der Lernfähigkeit in der sozialen Umwelt*. Münich: Kinder Verlag.
Mann, A., A. Harrell, & M. Hunt. 1976. *A review of Headstart research since 1969*. Washington, D.C.: Social Research Group.
Manning, F. & C. Feyerabend. 1976. Cigarette smoking and fetal breathing movements. *British Journal of Obstetrics and Gynaecology* 83:262–70.
Mantell, C. 1964. Smoking in pregnancy: The role played by carbonic anhydrase. *New Zealand Medical Journal* 63:601–603.
Martin, J. & R. Becker. 1970. The effects of nicotine administration in utero upon activity in the rat. *Psychonomic Science* 19:59–60.
Martin, J., D. Martin, C. Lund, & A. Streissguth. 1977. Maternal alcohol ingestion and cigarette smoking and their effects on newborn conditioning. *Alcoholism: Clinical and Experimental Results*, 1:243–47.
Matas, L., R. A. Arend, & L. A. Soufe. 1978. Continuity of adaptation in the second year: The relationship between quality of attachment and later competence. *Child Development* 49:547–56.
Mau, G. 1976. Smoking and the fetus. *Lancet* 1:972.
Maudry, M. & M. Nekula. 1939. Social relations between children of the same age during the first two years of life. *Journal of Genetic Psychology* 54:193–215.
Maynard, J. F. 1979. *Infant perception of auditory-visual synchrony*. Unpublished master's thesis, Urbana: University of Illinois.
Meredith, H. 1975. Relation between tobacco smoking of pregnant women and body size of their progeny: A compilation and synthesis of published studies. *Human Biology* 47:451–72.
Meyer, M., B. Jonas, & J. Tonascia. 1976. Perinatal events associated with maternal smoking during pregnancy. *American Journal of Epidemeology* 103:464–76.
Miller, H., K. Hassanein, & P. Hensleigh. 1976. Fetal growth retardation in relation to maternal smoking and weight gain in pregnancy. *American Journal of Obstetrics and Gynaecology* 1:55–60.

Money, J., J. G. Hampson, & J. L. Hampson. 1957. Imprinting and the establishment of gender role. *Archives of Neurology and Psychology* 77:333–36.
Moore, T. 1975. Exclusive early mothering and its alternatives: The outcome to adolescence. *Scnadinavian Journal of Psychology* 16:255–72.
Morgan, G. A. & H. N. Ricciutti. 1969. Infants' responses to strangers during the first year. In B. M. Foss, ed., *Determinants of Infant Behavior*, vol. 1. London: Methuen Press.
Moskowitz, D., J. Schwarz, & D. Corsini. 1977. Initiating day care at three years of age: Effects on attachment. *Child Development* 48:1271–76.
Mulcahy, R., I. Murphy, & F. Martin. 1970. Placental changes and maternal weight in smoking and nonsmoking mothers. *American Journal of Obstetrics and Gynaecology* 106:703–4.
Murphy, J. & R. Mulcahy. 1971. The effect of age, parity, and cigarette smoking on baby weight. *American Journal of Obstetrics and Gynaecology* 111:22–25.
Naeye, R. 1978. Relationship of cigarette smoking to congenital anomalies and perinatal death. *American Journal of Pathology* 90:289–93.
Naeye, R., W. Harkness, & J. Otts. 1977. Abruptio placentae and perinatal death: A prospective study. *American Journal of Obstetrics and Gynaecology* 128:740–46.
Naeye, R. L., B. Ladis, & J. S. Drage. 1976. Sudden infant death syndrome: A prospective study. *American Journal of Diseases of Children* 130:1207–1210.
National Academy of Sciences. 1976. *Toward a National Policy for Children and Families*. Washington, D.C.: National Academy of Sciences.
Nelson, K. 1973. Structure and strategy in learning to talk. *Monographs of the Society for Research in Child Development* 38:1–2, no. 149.
Nelson, K. 1977. First steps in language acquisition. *Journal of the American Academy of Child Psychiatry* 16:563–83.
Newcombe, R. 1976. Cigarette smoking in pregnancy. *British Medical Journal* 2:755.
Nichols, P. 1977. Minimal brain dysfunction: Association with perinatal complication. Paper presented at the biennial meeting of the Society for Research in Child Development, March 1977, New Orleans.
Nicolich, L. M. 1977. Beyond sensorimotor intelligence: Assessment of symbolic maturity through analysis of pretend play. *Merrill-Palmer Quarterly* 23:89–99.
Nie, N., C. Hull, J. Jenkins, K. Steinbrenner, & D. Dent. 1975. *Statistical Package for the Social Sciences*. New York: McGraw-Hill.

Niswander, K. & M. Gordon. 1972. *The Women and Their Pregnancies*. Philadelphia: W. B. Saunders.

Nymand, G. 1974. Maternal smoking and immunity. *Lancet* 2:1379–80.

O'Lane, J. 1963. Some fetal effects of maternal cigarette smoking. *Obstetrics and Gynaecology* 22:181–84.

Olds, D. 1980. Improving formal services for mothers and children. In J. Garbarino and H. Stocking, eds., *Protecting Children from Abuse and Neglect: Creating and Maintaining Family Support Systems*. San Francisco: Jossey-Bass.

Oster, H. S. 1975. Color perception in ten-week-old infants. Paper presented at the meeting of the Society for Research in Child Development, April 1975, Denver.

Overton, W. F. & J. P. Jackson. 1973. The representation of imagined objects in action sequences: A developmental study. *Child Development* 44:309–14.

Paine, R. S. 1976. The contribution of developmental neurology to child psychiatry. In E. N. Rexford, L. W. Sander, & T. Shapiro, eds., *Infant Psychiatry: A New Synthesis*. New Haven: Yale University Press.

Palmgren, B., T. Wahlen, & B. Wallander. 1973. Toxemia and cigarette smoking during pregnancy. *Acta. Obstet. Gynecol. Scand.* 52:183–185.

Parke, R. D. 1978. Perspectives on father-infant interaction. In J. D. Osofsky, ed., *Handbook of Infant Development*. New York: Wiley.

Parke, R. D. & S. O'Leary. 1976. Family interaction in the newborn period: Some findings, some observations, and some unresolved issues. In K. Riegel & J. Meacham, eds., *The Developing Individual in a Changing World*. Vol. 2, *Social and Environmental Issues*. The Hague: Mouton.

Parmelee, A. H. & A. Haber. 1973. Who is the "risk infant?" *Clinical Obstetrics and Gynecology* 16:396–387.

Pedersen, F. A. & K. S. Robson. 1969. Father participation in infancy. *American Journal of Orthopsychiatry* 39:466–472.

Peterson, W., K. Morese, & D. Kaltreida. 1965. Smoking and prematurity: A preliminary report based on study of 7,740 Caucasians. *Obstetrics and Gynaecology* 26:775–779.

Piaget, J. 1951. *Play, dreams, and imitation in childhood*. C. Gattegno & F. N. Hodgson, trans. New York: Norton.

Piaget, J. 1952. *The Origins of Intelligence in Children*. M. Cooke, trans. New York: International Universities Press.

Portnoy, F. & C. Simmons. 1978. Day care and attachment. *Child Development* 49:239–242.

Prentice, N. & J. Bieri. 1970. Intellectual development of culturally deprived children in a day care program: A follow-up study. Paper presented at the meeting of the American Orthopsychiatric Association, March 1970, San Francisco.

Protestos, C. D., R. G. Carpenter, P. B. McWeeny, & J. L. Emery. 1973. Obstetric and perinatal histories of children who died unexpectedly. *Archives of Diseases in Childhood* 48:835–841.

Provence, S. & R. Lipton. 1961. *Infants in Institutions*. New York: International University Press.

Purpura, D. P. 1975. Neuronal migration and dendritic differentiation: Normal and aberrant development of human cerebral cortex. In Mead Johnson Symposium on Perinatal and Developmental Medicine, no. 6: *Biological and Clinical Aspects of Brain Development* 13–27.

Radin, N. 1973. Observed paternal behaviors as antecedents of intellectual functioning in young boys. *Developmental Psychology* 8:369–376.

Ragozin, A. 1977. Attachment behavior of day care and home reared children in a laboratory setting. Paper presented at the biennial meeting of the Society for Research in Child Development, March 1977, New Orleans.

Ramey, C. & F. Campbell. 1977. The prevention of developmental retardation in high-risk children. In P. Mittler, ed., *Research to Practice in Mental Retardation*, vol. 1. *Care and Intervention*. Baltimore: University Park Press.

Ramey, C. & J. Mills. 1975. Mother-infant interaction patterns as a function of rearing conditions. Paper presented at the meeting of the Society for Research in Child Development, April, Denver.

Ramey, C. & B. Smith. 1976. Assessing the intellectual consequences of early intervention with high-risk infants. *American Journal of Mental Deficiency* 81:318–324.

Rebelsky, F. & C. Hanks. 1971. Fathers' verbal interaction with infants in the first three months of life. *Child Development* 42:63–68.

Reinke, W. & M. Henderson. 1966. Smoking and prematurity in the presence of other variables. *Archives of Environmental Health* 12:600–606.

Rhead, W. 1977. Smoking and SIDS. *Pediatrics* 59:791–792.

Rheingold, H. L. 1969. The effect of a strange environment on the behaviour of infants. In B. M. Foss, ed., *Determinants of Infant Behavior*, vol. 4. London: Methuen.

Rheingold, H. L. 1971. *Some visual determinants of smiling in infants*. Unpublished manuscript, University of North Carolina at Chapel Hill.

Rheingold, H. L. 1973. Independent behavior of the human infant. In *Minnesota Symposia on Child Psychology*, vol. 7. Minneapolis: University of Minnesota Press.

Rheingold, H. L. & C. O. Eckerman. 1971. Fear of the stranger: A cultural examination. Paper presented at the meetings of the Society for Research in Child Development, April 1971, Minneapolis.

Rheingold, H. L. & C. O. Eckerman. 1973. Fear of the stranger: A critical examination. In H. W. Reese, ed., *Advances in Child Development and Behavior*, vol. 8. New York: Academic Press.

Rheingold, H., J. Gewirtz, & H. Ross. 1959. Social conditioning of vocalizations in the infant. *Journal of Comparative and Physiological Psychology* 52:68–73.

Ricciuti, H. 1974. Fear and development of social attachments in the first year of life. In M. Lewis and L. A. Rosenblum, eds., *The Origins of Human Behavior: Fear*. New York: Wiley.

Richmond, J. 1979. *Healthy People: The Surgeon General's Report on Health Promotion and Disease Prevention*. U.S. Department of Health, Education, and Welfare, Public Health Service.

Riegel, K. 1972. Developmental psychology and society. In J. Nesselroade and H. Reese, eds., *Life-Span Psychology: Methodological Issues*. New York: Academic Press.

Riegel, K. 1975. Structure and transformation in modern intellectual history. In K. Riegel & J. Rosenwald, eds., *Structure and Transformation: Developmental and Historical Aspects*. New York: Wiley.

Ringler, N., J. Kennell, R. Jarvella, B. Navijosky, & M. Klaus. 1975. Mothers-to-child speech at two years—effects of early postnatal contacts. *Behavioral Pediatrics* 86:141–44.

The Robert Wood Johnson Foundation Special Report. 1978. No. 2.

Robinson, H. & N. Robinson. 1971. Longitudinal development of very young children in a comprehensive day care program: The first two years. *Child Development* 42:1673–83.

Roopnarine, J. & M. Lamb. 1978. The effects of day care on attachment and exploratory behavior in a strange situation. *Merrill-Palmer Quarterly* 24:85–95.

Rosenblatt, J. 1970. Views on the onset and maintenance of maternal behavior in the rat. In *Development and Evolution of Behavior*. San Francisco: Freeman.

Rovee, C. K. & D. T. Rovee. 1969. Conjugate reinforcement of infant exploratory behavior. *Journal of Experimental Child Psychology* 8:1–8.

Rubenstein, J. L. 1967. Maternal attentiveness and subsequent exploratory behavior. *Child Development* 38:1089–1100.

Rubenstein, J. L. & C. Howes. 1976. The effects of peers on toddler interaction with mothers and toys. *Child Development* 47:597–605.

Ruff, H. A. & H. G. Birch. 1974. Infant visual fixation: The effects of concentricity, curvilinearity, and number of directions. *Journal of Experimental Child Psychology* 17:460–473.

Rush, D., Z. Stein & M. Susser. 1980a. A randomized controlled trial of prenatal nutritional supplementation on New York City. *Pediatrics* 65:683–97.

Rush, D., Z. Stein & M. Susser. 1980b. Diet and pregnancy: A randomized controlled trial of prenatal nutritional supplementation. *Birth Defects* 16: in press.

Russell, C. 1974. Transition to parenthood: Problems and qualifications. *Journal of Marriage and the Family* 36:294–301.

Russell, C., R. Taylor, & C. Law. 1968. Smoking in pregnancy, maternal blood pressure, pregnancy outcome, baby weight and growth, and other related factors: A prospective study. *British Journal of the Society for Preventive Medicine* 22:119–26.

Rutter, M. 1970. Psychological development—predictions from infancy. *Journal of Child Psychology and Psychiatry* 11:49–62.

Ryan, J. 1974. Early language development. Towards a communicational analysis. In M. P. M. Richards, ed., *The Integration of a Child into a Social World*. New York: Cambridge University Press.

Salapatek, P. 1968. Visual scanning of geometric figures by the human newborn. *Journal of Comparative and Physiological Psychology* 66:247–258.

Salapatek, P., A. G. Bechtold, & E. W. Bushnell. 1976. Infant visual acuity as a function of viewing distance. *Child Development* 47:860–863.

Sameroff, A. J. & M. J. Chandler. 1975. Reproductive risk and the continuum of caretaking casualty. In F. D. Horowitz, M. Hetherington, S. Scarr-Salapatek, & G. Siegel, eds., *Review of Child Development Research*, vol. 4. Chicago: University of Chicago Press.

Saunders, M. 1972. Some aspects of the effects of day care on infants' emotional and personality development. Unpublished doctoral dissertation, University of North Carolina.

Schaffer, H. R. 1966. The onset of fear of strangers and the incongruity hypothesis. *Journal of Child Psychology and Psychiatry* 7:95–106.

Schaffer, H. R. 1971. *The Growth of Sociability*. Harmondsworth, England: Penguin.

Schaffer, H. R. & P. E. Emerson. 1964. The Development of Social Attachments in Infancy. *Monographs of the Society for Research in Child Development*, vol. 29(3, serial no. 94).

Schneirla, T., J. Rosenblatt, & E. Tobach. 1963. Maternal behavior in the cat. In J. Rheingold, ed., *Maternal Behavior in Mammals*. New York: Wiley.

Schoeneck, W. 1941. Cigarette smoking in pregnancy. *New York Journal of Medicine* 41:119–126.

Schwartz, M. 1975. *Visual Shape Perception in Early Infancy*. Unpublished doctoral dissertation, Monash University.

Siegel, E., K. Bauman & E. Schaefer. 1980. Hospital and home support during infancy: Impact on maternal attachment, child abuse and neglect, and health care utilization. *Pediatrics*: in press.

Simpson, W. 1957. A preliminary report on cigarette smoking and the incidence of prematurity. *American Journal of Obstetrics and Gynaecology* 73:808–15.

Sinclair, H. 1970. The transition from sensory-motor behavior to symbolic activity. *Interchange* 1:119–26.

Snow, C. E. 1977. The development of conversations between mothers and babies. *Journal of Child Language* 4:1–22.

Sontag, L. & R. Wallace. 1935. The effect of cigarette smoking during pregnancy upon the fetal heart rate. *American Journal of Obstetrics and Gynaecology* 29:77–83.

Sousa, P., F. Baros, R. Cazalle, R. Begeres, G. Pinheiro, S. Menezes, & L. Arruda. 1974. Attachment and lactation. Presented at Pediatria XIV: Nutrition, Toxicology and Pharmacology, Buenos Aires, Argentina.

Spelke, E. S. 1978. *Perceiving bimodally specified events.* Paper presented at the International Conference on Infant Studies, March, 1978, Providence, Rhode Island.

Spira, A., N. Spira, J. Goujard, & D. Schwartz. 1975. Smoking during pregnancy and placental weight. *Journal of Perinatal Medicine* 3:237–241.

Spitz, R. A. 1945. Hospitalism: An inquiry into the genesis of psychiatric conditions in early childhood. *Psychoanalytic Study of the Child* 1:53–74.

Sroufe, L. A. 1977. *Knowing and Enjoying Your Baby.* Englewood Cliffs, N.J. Prentice-Hall.

Sroufe, L. A. 1978. Attachment and the roots of competence. *Human Nature*, October, 1978, 50–59.

Sroufe, L. A. 1979. Socioemotional development. In J. Osofsky, ed., *Handbook of Infant Development.* New York: Wiley.

Sroufe, L. A. & E. Waters. 1977. Attachment as an organizational construct. *Child Development* 48:1184–1199.

Sroufe, L. A., E. Waters, & L. Matas. 1974. Contextual determinants of infant affective response. In M. Lewis & L. Rosenblum, eds., *The Origins of Fear.* New York: Wiley.

Standley, K., A. Soule, S. Copans, & R. Klein. 1978. Multidimensional sources of infant temperament. *Genetic Psychology Monographs* 98:203–232.

Steinschneider, A. 1976. Implications of the sudden infant death syndrome for the study of sleep in infancy. Paper presented at a symposium on crib death at meetings of the American Psychological Association, September, Washington, D.C.

Stern, D. 1974a. The goal and functions of mother-infant play. *Journal of the American Academy of Child Psychiatry* 13:402–421.

Stern, D. 1974b. Mother and infant at play: The dyadic interaction involving facial, vocal, and gaze behaviors. In M. Lewis & L. A. Rosenblum, eds., *The Effect of the Infant on Its Caregiver*. New York: Wiley.

Stern, D. 1977. *The First Relationship*. Cambridge: Harvard Univ. Press.

Stott, L. H. & R. S. Ball. 1965. Infant and Preschool Mental Tests: Review and Evaluation. Monographs for the Society of Research in Child Development 30, no. 101.

Strauss, M. S. & L. B. Cohen. 1978. Infant immediate and delayed memory for perceptual dimensions. Unpublished manuscript, University of Illinois.

Sutton-Smith, B. & B. G. Rosenberg. 1970. *The Sibling*. New York: Holt, Rinehart & Winston.

Terman, L. M. & M. A. Merrill. 1973. *The Stanford-Binet Intelligence Scale*. New York: Houghton Mifflin.

Thoman, E., V. N. Miano, & M. P. Freese. 1976. The role of respiratory instability in SIDS. Paper presented in symposium on crib death at meetings of the American Psychological Association, September 1976.

Thomas, A., S. Chess, & H. Brich. 1968. *Temperament and Behavior Disorders in Children*. New York: New York University Press.

Thomas, H. 1970. Psychological assessment instruments for use with human infants. *Merrill-Palmer Quarterly* 16:179–224.

Todd, G. & B. Palmer. 1968. Social reinforcement of infant babbling. *Child Development* 39:591–596.

Tronick, E. & T. Brazelton. 1975. Clinical uses of the Brazelton Neonatal Assessment. In B. Z. Friedlauder, G. M. Sterritt & G. E. Kirk, eds., *Exceptional Infant 3: Assessment and Intervention*. New York: Bruner/Mazel.

Underwood, P., K. Kesler, J. O'Lane, & D. Callagan. 1967. Parental smoking empirically related to pregnancy outcome. *Obstetrics and Gynaecology* 29:1–8.

Uzgiris, I. 1976. Organization of sensorimotor intelligence. In M. Lewis, Ed., *Origins of Intelligence*. New York: Plenum.

Valentine, C. W. 1913–1914. The colour perception and colour preferences of an infant during its fourth and eighth months. *British Journal of Psychology* 6:363–86.

Vaughn, B., E. Waters, B. Egeland, & L. A. Sroufe. 1979. Individual differences in infant-mother attachment at 12 and 18 months: Stability and change in families under stress. *Child Development* 50:971–75.

Vincze, M. 1971. The social contacts of infants and young children reared together. *Early Child Development and Care* 1:99–109.

Vurpillot, E., J. Ruel, & A. Castrec. 1977. L'organisation perceptive chez le nourrisson: Réponse au tout ou á ses éléments? *Bulletin de Psychologie* 327:396–405.

Vygotsky, L. 1967. Play and its role in the mental development of the child. *Soviet Psychology* 5:6–18.

Waldrop, M., R. Bell, B. McLaughlin, & C. Halverson. 1978. Newborn minor physical anomalies predict short attention span, peer aggression and impulsivity at age 3. *Science* 199:563–65.

Wallace, A. F. C. 1961. *Culture and Personality*. New York: Random House.

Wallach, M. A. & N. Kogan. 1965. *Modes of Thinking in Young Children*. New York: Holt, Rinehart & Winston.

Wallston, B. 1973. The effects of maternal employment on children. *Journal of Child Psychology and Psychiatry* 14:81–95.

Waters, E. 1978. The reliability and stability of individual differences in infant-mother attachment. *Child Development* 49:483–494.

Waters, E., J. Wippman, & L. A. Sroufe. 1979. Attachment, positive affect, and competence in the peer group: Two studies in construct validation. *Child Development* 50:821–829.

Watson, J. 1966. The development and generalization of contingency awareness in early infancy: Some hypotheses. *Merrill-Palmer Quarterly* 12:123–135.

Watson, J. S. 1972. Smiling, cooing, and "the game." *Merrill-Palmer Quarterly*, 12:123–135.

Watson, M. W. & K. W. Fischer. 1977. A developmental sequence of agent use in late infancy. *Child Development* 48:828–836.

Weisberg, P. 1963. Social and nonsocial conditioning of infant vocalizations. *Child Development* 34:377–388.

Weisler, A. & R. B. McCall. 1976. Exploration and play: Resume and redirection. *American Psychologist* 31:492–508.

White, B. L. & J. C. Watts. 1973. *Experience and Environment*. Englewood Cliffs, N.J.: Prentice-Hall.

White, R. 1959. Motivation reconsidered: The concept of competence. *Psychological Review* 66:297–333.

Winters, M. 1973. The relationship of time of initial breastfeeding to success of breastfeeding. Nursing master's thesis, University of Washington.

Yang, R. & H. Moss. 1978. Neonatal precursors of infant behavior. *Developmental Psychology* 14:607–613.

Yogman, M. W. 1977. The goals and structure of face-to-face interaction between infants and fathers. Paper presented at the Biennial Meeting of the Society for Research in Child Development, March 1977, New Orleans.

Zabriskie, J. 1963. Effects of cigarette smoking during pregnancy. *Obstetrics and Gynaecology* 21:405–411.

Zelazo, P. R. 1980. The year old infant: A period of major cognitive change. In T. Bever, ed., *Dips in Developmental Curves*. Hillsdale, N.J.: L. Erlbaum Associates.
Zelazo, P. R. & R. B. Kearsley. 1977. Functional play: Evidence for a cognitive metamorphosis in the year old infant. Paper presented at the biennial meeting of the Society for Research in Child Development, March 1977, New Orleans.
Zelazo, P. R. & R. B. Kearsley. 1980. The emergence of functional play in infants: Evidence for a major cognitive transition. *Journal of Applied Developmental Psychology*, in press.
Zigler, E. & I. L. Child. 1968. Socialization. In G. Lindzey & E. Aronson, eds., *The Handbook of Social Psychology*, vol. 3. Reading, Mass.: Addison-Wesley.

Bei Fragen zur Produktsicherheit wenden Sie sich bitte an:
If you have any questions regarding product safety,
please contact:

Walter de Gruyter GmbH
Genthiner Straße 13
10785 Berlin
productsafety@degruyterbrill.com